Stories from Italian Forensic Psychiatric Hospitals

Jacopo Santambrogio

Stories from Italian Forensic Psychiatric Hospitals

palgrave
macmillan

Jacopo Santambrogio
ASST Brianza
Presidio "G. Corberi" and RSD "Beato Papa Giovanni XXIII"
Limbiate, Italy

ISBN 978-3-031-61128-5 ISBN 978-3-031-61129-2 (eBook)
https://doi.org/10.1007/978-3-031-61129-2

This Palgrave Macmillan imprint is published by the registered company Springer Nature Switzerland AG.
The registered company address is: Gewerbestrasse 11, 6330 Cham, Switzerland

Paper in this product is recyclable.

Foreword

Psychiatry. There is not just one psychiatry, but two. There is the psychiatry that considers psychopathological experiences as being the consequence of neurobiological deficits, ignoring the patients' interpersonal and social problems. Then there is the psychiatry that considers these experiences as being caused by a combination of factors, biological, psychological, and social. These two approaches have eventuated in two radically different methods of engaging with those suffering from a mental illness: the first considers patients with scientific detachment, as if analysing and describing a diseased body or, to be more precise, a diseased brain, without attributing any importance at all to their interiority, to their emotional relations; the second probes the innermost recesses of these patients' minds, their expectations and their anguish, their sadness, their relationships, in order to acquire knowledge of their ways of being, and of their disorders, in the context of a relationship based on trust. Only by laying aside all prejudice is it possible to achieve this type of intimacy with the psychically ill; they must be treated with respect, accepted as they are, in all their alterity, their "otherness", their ardent humanity, their suffering. In spite of their problems, they have the same expectations and hopes as we more fortunate beings. This is the psychiatry that Jacopo Santambrogio has applied in his reflections on the transformation of the Forensic Psychiatric Hospitals into Residences for the Execution of Protective Measures (known as REMS).

In Italian mental hospitals, the first type of psychiatry predominated; the living conditions were terrible and the treatments worse, even twenty-five years after the discovery of anti-psychotics (the first, Largactil, came onto the market in 1952), and would have remained so if Franco Basaglia,[1] working first in Gorizia and later in Trieste, had not brought about an incredible revolution in the comprehension of the social roots of madness, demonstrating that treatment of psychotic disorders could not be reconciled with life in mental hospitals where the patient was devastated by indifference and lack of humanity. The reform of 1978 introduced the closure of these institutions (and consequently of the Forensic Psychiatric Hospitals where perpetrators of crimes, affected by mental illnesses, were confined) and laid the foundations for a new form of psychiatry which began to play a role in general hospitals and the local healthcare services.

This book throws light on the intolerable violence of the Italian Forensic Psychiatric Hospitals, where the living conditions were even worse, more terrifying, and inhuman than those of the civil institutions. He has described the indescribable in his accounts of the conditions in which the inmates of Barcellona Pozzo di Gotto, Montelupo Fiorentino, and Reggio Emilia lived or, to be more precise, struggled to survive. Reading these pages, it is difficult to imagine how it was possible to eliminate this violence and render the new structures operative. The book provides a preliminary overview of the essential aspects of these structures and their importance from the psychopathological and human standpoints.

What makes this book so interesting, even more than the technical accounts, are the descriptions of the atrocious suffering of the inmates confined to these Forensic Psychiatric Hospitals and the discovery of their unexpected and surprising capacity for self-expression and creativity. These stories, elicited with rare sensibility and care, make disturbing reading and are very hard to forget.

The question that arises from the book, and it is a distressing question, is this: how did doctors and nurses, health service directors, and

---

[1] Franco Basaglia (1924–1980) spearheaded the reform of legislation on mental health in Italy, contributing significantly to the closure of the mental hospitals. He is considered to be one of the most influential Italian psychiatrists of the twentieth century.

politicians manage to stand by and allow such inhuman conditions to exist without rebelling, accepting responsibility? How could they have been so indifferent to human suffering, so inert?

Building on a painstaking labour of interpreting and deciphering the innermost depths of these lives, particularly the emotions lacerated by immense suffering, and exploring the extreme confines of anguish and desperation, including the death wish, this book reveals the complexity and depths of madness that does not differentiate between the innocent and those who have committed crimes.

Jacopo Santambrogio, writing in a limpid style that highlights his passion for the subject, probes the hidden and sometimes unfathomable aspects of madness while respecting the patients' dignity and liberty of expression and accepting that anti-psychotics and social therapy are co-adjutants and can only function if there is dialogue with a person who listens, empathizes, and participates emotionally. These were the methods promoted by Franco Basaglia, who pioneered a new approach to mental health and brought about the revolution that led to the closure of the mental hospitals and so indirectly of the Forensic Psychiatric Hospitals. These methods made it possible, then as now, to familiarize with the knowledge and therapies of the psychiatry based on anthropological and interpretative foundations that emerge so clearly from these pages. The book, with its detailed descriptions of the interiority and sensibility of patients who spent their days buried alive in the Forensic Psychiatric Hospitals and who now mostly reside in the REMS that are radically different from a relational and therapeutic standpoint, provides the reader with a fresh understanding of the psychopathological and clinical, phenomenological and psychodynamical aspects of madness.

This book provides evidence of just how much humanity survives even in the psychically ill who have committed crimes, humanity that psychiatric naturalism has never succeeded in acknowledging in all its dilemmatic suffering. Taking the masterfully reconstructed life stories of several of the inmates of the Forensic Psychiatric Hospitals as a starting point, the book discusses the major themes of a humane and interpretative psychiatry that significantly expands its semantic boundaries.

The author addresses these themes with passion and dedication, a rare propensity for listening and dialogue, and an extraordinarily profound capacity for interpretation and originality of thought, guiding the reader to an understanding of the roots of clinical psychiatry and of the psychiatry that is applied in the REMS, partly reducing the distance—which obviously cannot be eliminated—between the two forms. This is a book that sheds fresh light on the topic of knowledge and therapy in psychiatry, bearing constantly in mind its ethical foundations that are so essential to its being, formal and thematic declinations apart. As a book based on a vast knowledge of psychiatric theories and practices, and a rare background of clinical and psychotherapeutic experience, it is also of great interest from the didactical point of view. It is a book which provides information on a subject that has vastly overlapping cultural themes for readers interested in psychiatry and in the forensic and social sciences, a book that enriches the reader in the quest for the comprehension and acceptance of madness.

Eugenio Borgna is Director Emeritus of Psychiatry of the University Hospital Maggiore della Carità of Novara. He was one of the first psychiatrists in Italy to apply the theoretical principles of anthropo-analysis and phenomenological psychopathology to the study of mental illness. He has written many specialized texts on psychiatry, as well as books for a wider audience.

University Hospital Maggiore della Carità
Novara, Italy
Eugenio Borgna

Foreword

THE TRANSITION FROM THE FORENSIC PSYCHIATRIC HOSPITALS
TO THE RESIDENCES FOR THE EXECUTION OF SECURITY MEASURES

Opportunities for a change in the strategy for mental health treatment for persons who have committed crimes

Over the last few years, the subject of patients with mental disorders who have committed a crime has not only stimulated a significant degree of clinical and scientific interest among mental health professionals but has also caused increasing concern regarding the repercussions on the psychiatric services; both interest and concern are shared by magistrates, prison administrators, social service operators, and also by the public. What is the explanation for this reaction, which is spreading like wildfire and is involving such diverse groups of people?

Probably the explanation lies in the progressive acceleration of correlated phenomena that on the one hand have seen the development of new needs and, on the other, of critical issues that have caused—and are still causing—professionals and non-professionals to raise questions to which there are no easy answers: e.g., how should the perpetrator of a crime who is suffering from psychopathological disorders be considered? When does antisocial behaviour become an illness? what constitutes being *a danger to society*? What courses of treatment/rehabilitation does the Health Service offer under these conditions? Assuming such courses are available and are followed to the letter, what are the possibilities of being cured? What is the toll of the requests for social control that are unloaded on psychiatry and the judiciary at the present?

These questions are being considered outside the sphere of mental health more frequently than before, and they throw light not only on the organizational scenarios of the Health Services, but also on social concerns. Increasingly often, also, there are consequences from the *media circus*, where the line between scientific information and press manipulation to whip up public opinion becomes very thin indeed.

The phenomena to which I am referring are diachronically connected to a number of factors: firstly, to the strong ideological pressure surrounding the closure of the Forensic Psychiatric Hospitals (FPHs) and the preparation of the relevant actuation norms; secondly and subsequently, to the debate among operators—in which public opinion played a part—regarding the implementation of the new structures, the Residences for the Execution of Security Measures (known as REMS), designated to substitute the FPHs and which were completely new in every aspect (as no experimentation had been done with these structures there was no evidence as to their feasibility or efficacy); and lastly, to the hands-on stage and the heterogeneous interpretation that psychiatrists, judiciary, and public opinion would make of it.

These rather uninformed controversies between mental health operators and other professionals or between the former and the judiciary were kept alive for a long period of time by this sequence of events that were often tinged with the anxiety typical of revolutionary innovations and the uncertainty of an empirical approach which, it must be said, was hardly influenced at all by scientific evidence from the rest of the world. Indeed, they reinforced the various non-specific requests for social controls that are difficult to satisfy at the best of times in the absence of concrete data, and often are only sparked off by emotive reactions.

At national and regional levels, the legislation regarding persons committing crimes while affected by mental disorders has resulted in stimulating debates between scientific and professional communities, as well as the constitution of work groups, all of which continue to offer food for thought both from a clinical and an organizational point of view. One example of this is the sharing of documentation between the Department of Mental Health and the Judiciary of the Lombardy region in Italy, which lays the basis for an area of cooperation essential for monitoring the placement of these persons, not only in the REMS but also in traditional prisons which were immediately affected by the difficulties deriving from the new norms.

In recent years, within the Department of Mental Health (and indeed the Department of Mental Health and Addiction as is the case in many Italian regions), the planning of processes for the development—and the gradual activation—of experimental projects to replace the FPHs, and aiming at reinforcing the clinical area dedicated to dealing with the psychically ill who have committed a crime, tends to respond to two specific categories of patients in particular:

1. Patients with time still to serve of their custodial sentences, on probation or under house arrest, etc.;
2. FPH patients who have already served their sentences and are undergoing rehabilitation and reintegration into the community.

Regarding the first case, the law that has provided for the realization of the REMS to replace the FPHs appears adequate, at least superficially, to respond to the organizational aspects for the containment of the more complex psychopathological cases and those at risk of relapse; the main problem, however, lies in the number of available structures and the diversity of the requirements, in terms of therapy and rehabilitation, of the prospective inmates who have committed a crime. The issue therefore is to match the characteristics of the inmates, i.e., the type of crime they have committed and the mental disorders afflicting them, with the structures and corresponding therapeutic and rehabilitative facilities.

For those patients belonging to the second group, i.e., the FPH inmates who have completed their custodial sentence, none of the highly integrated solutions described at length in the law regarding the closure of the FPHs, or discussed from an operational point of view by the Departments of Mental Health, seem to be available at the time of writing; a further complication lies in the fact that both the law and its actuation decrees are frequently referred to in regional norms and operational documents such as guidelines and the Diagnostic and Therapeutic Care Pathways.

Moreover, again at the time of writing, the Departments of Mental Health appear to function on the basis of a substantially administrative mandate, and this, taken together with the current organizational structure, does not seem to provide them with access to adequate instruments and clinical support to deal with patients at risk of suffering relapses as well as the presence of cases of social dangerousness that have not been completely restored to health in spite of the treatment and rehabilitation courses.

The current approach is based on institutional frameworks which continue to be bound to general and sporadic measures or guided prevalently by the need to safeguard the local public: this is done by creating circuits—mainly non-specific and indistinct—that more than anything else underline the ever-growing need and criticality for beds and the quest for procedures usually of a restraining nature, forcibly solicited by the pressure for social control from the locality.

This approach tends to recreate a type of *dedicated psychiatric community* for people affected by this type of pathology (frequently significantly psychopathologically comorbid and not infrequently accompanied by a prevalence of mixed aspects characteristic of antisocial personality disorders with drug abuse and previous premature vulnerability) in a single therapeutic rehabilitation environment. Instead of adopting proven clinical rules and procedures, these *communities* tend to be simply containment centres with little diversification. As a result, the solution offered by the prison structure, focused as it is on social control and by definition non-specific, is seen as approaching the clinical solutions to social control that are currently being experimented by the Social Health Departments; this facilitates the possibility of prisons being used as transition hubs or as permanent solutions for those patients for whom it has not been possible to find a bed in the REMS, or who are too antisocial for the treatment available in the REMS to guarantee protection against their social dangerousness.

Therefore, over the last two years the context has generated, in some cases inappropriately, reformatory guidelines with proposals to modify national legislation or has given rise to experiments at the regional level outside the institutions that do not conform to the national law and pay scarce attention to the procedures that should reallocate the available residential resources and specific treatment and/or rehabilitation courses. Notwithstanding these trends, however, it must be said that while the construction of new, specialized structures to house and care for patients who have committed crimes is unlikely to be completed in the short term, the role assumed by the prison circuit is revealing similarly worrisome scenarios as to sustainability both by the Prison Administration and by the Mental Health Department.

Another issue is the lack of concrete data regarding those patients who, once discharged, have suffered a relapse and of information regarding the qualitative-quantitative efficacy of the alternative measures. It is extremely difficult to make concrete proposals for new solutions in the absence of assessment studies regarding the patients or detailed studies of the various courses of therapy and rehabilitation designed for the different sub-populations with the objective of better identifying the costs/benefits of the programmes and define valid indicators for a more accurate selection of patients based on their psychopathological characteristics and penal profiles.

Aside from these problems, and on a more general note, it must be said that in the experience of the Departments of Mental Health, the onerous issue of territorial responsibility for those patients who have committed a crime is still a sort of niche for a chosen few. It is too far removed from the daily clinical reality and is perceived by the operators as a clinical area to be managed, mostly or even exclusively, by the *medicine/prison psychiatry* circuits or by an institution resembling a reformed version of the FPH but continues to be without strong and stable links to the territorial activities of the local Department of Mental Health.

The transformation that Italian healthcare is currently undergoing can cultivate and induce important changes in the current scenario as, starting with the allocation of the healthcare for these patients to the Regional Healthcare Services, it must provide for the gradual absorption of penitentiary and forensic medicine/psychiatry into the sphere of the basic activities of the Department of Mental Health. Take for example the mental health services provided in prison, above all prevention of self-harming, as well as the acknowledgement of the prisoners' right to treatment and the central role of the public psychiatrist as a forensic expert.

The Department of Mental Health must therefore assume responsibility for the activities that previously were allocated to the penitentiary healthcare system, and this cannot be limited to psychiatric support in prison but must include direct management of alternative security measures (house arrest, probation at home or in psychiatric institutions, release on experimental licence, etc.) and the creation of a model of forensic psychiatry updated for healthcare services instead of the external expert/consultant chosen by the magistrate.

To conclude, the norms dictating the closure of the FPHs have led not only to the creation of alternative residential structures (the REMS), but also to the (somewhat arduous) development of a support network extended to include antisociality and, most importantly, to the pathologies that presently contribute to it, such as personality disorders and the so-called *double diagnosis* for mental disorders and drug abuse. Although there is still plenty of room for doubt in terms of activation of specific *treatment courses at territorial level* and at least potentially, from a practical standpoint more attention to this constantly increasing phenomenon can at least partially restructure the operational psychiatric model created in Italy in the 1980s.

It is to be hoped that significant investments will be allocated to providing training for Department of Mental Health operators in the change in orientation of the new clinical practices and, at the same time, guarantee not only the acquisition of new specialistic competences but also a necessary boost to the level of motivation so that their approach to this complex patient typology will be realistic and as complete as possible.

This book offers the reader a historical reconstruction of the events leading up to the closure of the FPHs and a detailed examination of clinical cases that were characteristic of these institutions. It is an attempt to contribute to a reordering of the considerations discussed here and opens the way to a gradual discovery of how the situation evolved. These stories provide an insight into how the inmates lived; they themselves may change but the gravity of the problems remains the same, and the present debate must be based on a reconstruction of the experiences gained in the past. If we are to understand future events, close attention must be paid to the very often distressing experiences of those who spent years of their lives in these psychiatric institutions.

Massimo Clerici is Full Professor of Psychiatry (MED-25) and Director of the Post-graduate School of Psychiatry of the University of Milano-Bicocca. He is also Director of the Department of Mental Health and Addiction of the Fondazione IRCCS San Gerardo dei Tintori, Monza, Italy.

Milano, Italy
Monza, Italy

Massimo Clerici

Preface to the English Edition

On May 13, 1978, the Basaglia Law, or Law 180/1978 as it is formally known, laid the basis for the closure of the Italian mental hospitals; Laws 9/2012 and 81/2014 formalized the closure of the Forensic Psychiatric Hospitals, institutions that had been operational since 1975.

In 2013 I was fortunate enough to obtain permission to visit the Forensic Psychiatric Hospitals before their closure with the photojournalist, Caterina Clerici. My objective was to document the state of the art of the facilities, the organizational aspects, and the care provided. I had the unique opportunity to talk with the inmates and to "see" the institutions through their voices. The picture I pieced together from their stories reflects the reality of these hospitals from 1975 to 2015, and I decided to compile a book with the material collected, to document this reality.

Why did I decide to have the book translated into English?

Firstly, I felt that an international audience of mental health professionals and people interested in psychiatry could be curious about the history of forensic psychiatric institutions in Italy; secondly I felt that an update about our forensic mental health system that has transited from Forensic Psychiatric Hospitals to a new system of Residencies for the Execution of Security Measures (known as REMS) could be of interest. This new model is specifically designed for forensic patients and is based on the community mental health system. In Italy, persons who suffer from psychic illness and have committed crimes now have new treatment pathways, focused on rehabilitation and recovery rather than institutionalization.

The English version also includes follow-up interviews with two of the original protagonists, "Fausto" and "Davide", both of whom now live in community settings oriented to rehabilitation where they experience more freedom and hope for the future.

I am an Italian psychiatrist, trained in phenomenology, psychiatry, and psychoanalysis, I have worked for 7 years in the field of rehabilitation for persons with severe mental illnesses and legal issues (Adele Bonolis AS.FRA. Foundation) and in Intellectual Disability and Autism residential facilities (Presidio G. Corberi and RSD Beato Papa Giovanni XXIII) that is now my my main job. Since my residency in psychiatry, I have developed a specific interest in forensic psychiatry and the history both of mental hospitals and of Forensic Psychiatric Hospitals.

This is a book of clinical psychiatry, based on interviews with mentally disturbed offenders and the mental health professionals who had them in care; the intention is to give an unbiased view of the Italian Forensic Psychiatric Hospitals, as opposed to that predominantly offered by journalistic and sociological literature. It gives voice to the people who lived in the institutions, rather than focusing on the institutions themselves and their organization as is often the case in scientific literature—a voice that, as psychiatrists, we must listen to with care.

Presidio "G. Corberi" and RSD "Beato Papa Giovanni XXIII", Limbiate (MB), Italy
Jacopo Santambrogio

Acknowledgments

Adele Bonolis AS.FRA. Foundation, founded by the Venerable Servant of God Adele Bonolis (1909–1980), is an Italian rehabilitation residential facility dedicated to severe mental health patients. The Foundation is accredited with the Lombardy Regional Health System and under contract with ATS Monza Brianza. It includes four communities of 20 patients each, some of them with legal issues and on probation. After Law 81/2014 AS.FRA. could be considered for some mentally ill offenders an alternative rehabilitative treatment compared to the custodial pathways in jails or in the Residencies for the Execution of Security Measure (REMS).

A special word of thanks is due to Adele Bonolis AS.FRA. Foundation and its president, dott. Alessandro Pirola, who supported the project and the cultural aims of this book.

Frances Anderson

Contents

1

Introduction

Trieste, January 2012. My journey of discovery into the world of Italy's Forensic Psychiatric Hospitals, the faces and stories of the inmates, started from the city where one of the country's most influential psychiatrists, Franco Basaglia, worked and studied. I was still a student with a few months to spare before starting a course of specialization in psychiatry at the University of Milano-Bicocca in Monza under the direction of Prof. Massimo Clerici, and I decided to pass the time following Basaglia's footsteps, visiting the places that have left an indelible mark on the history of Italian psychiatry. From the ex-psychiatric hospital of San Giovanni and the social co-operative Sartoria Sociale Lister, I was catapulted into the home of Dr. Giuseppe Dell'Acqua, who had studied under Franco Basaglia. Together with Dr. Franco Rotelli and a group of friends and colleagues, Dr. Dell'Acqua was writing a paper with the title, "Regarding the closure of Forensic Psychiatric Hospitals: the good intentions of a risky law" (*A proposito della chiusura dell'Ospedale Psichiatrico Giudiziario: le buone intenzioni di una legge pericolosa*).[1] The group was worried about

[1] Rotelli, F., Gallio, G., Dell'Acqua, P., Del Giudice, G., Carrino, L., Novello, M. et al. (2012). *A proposito della chiusura dell'Ospedale Psichiatrico Giudiziario: le buone intenzioni di una legge pericolosa.* https://www.lavoroculturale.org/reparto-agitati-3-a-proposito-della-chiusura-dellospedale-psichiatrico-giudiziario/franco-rotelli/2012/.

J. Santambrogio, *Stories from Italian Forensic Psychiatric Hospitals*,
https://doi.org/10.1007/978-3-031-61129-2_1

how the new, purely medical structures would manage to deal with *mad criminals*. At the time I had no idea of what a Forensic Psychiatric Hospital (FPH) really was, and the concepts of *mad criminals*, security measures, social danger were new to me, but my passion for psychiatry and its history spurred me on to ask questions as if I were a journalist reporting on a medical issue, and so I made my first approach to this area of psychiatry under Dr. Dell'Acqua's aegis. It was a delicate, and above all historical, moment. More than thirty years had passed since the approval of Law 180/833 of May 13, 1978, but finally major changes were afoot; the first, fundamental breakthrough in the closing of mental hospitals was achieved thanks to the experiences here in Trieste and Franco Basaglia's determination and obduracy.[2, 3, 4, 5, 6, 7, 8, 9]

Just three years earlier in 2009, Ignazio Marino, a senator of the Italian Republic who led a Parliamentary Commission of Inquiry into the efficacy and efficiency of the country's National Health Service, visited the Department of Mental Health in Trieste. In the same year, on August 4, a fifty-eight-year-old elementary school teacher, Francesco Mastrogiovanni, died in the hospital of Vallo della Lucania in Campania. He had been forcibly hospitalized by a compulsory mental health order (involuntary psychiatric commitment). His death after ninety-four hours bound to a bed, sedated and dehydrated, shocked the nation.[10] The Commission turned its attention to psychiatry and how it should be

---

[2] For a comprehensive introduction to the work and reforms of Franco Basaglia, see Foot, J. (2015). *The Man Who Closed the Asylums: Franco Basaglia and the Revolution in Mental Health Care.* Verso.

[3] Basaglia, F. (2010). *L'istituzione negata. Rapporto da un Ospedale psichiatrico.* Baldini Castoldi Dalai.

[4] Basaglia, F. (2000). *Conferenze Brasiliane.* Raffaello Cortina Editore.

[5] Basaglia, F. Ongaro Basaglia, F., Pirella, A., Taverna, S. (2008). Raffaello Cortina Editore.

[6] Basaglia, A. (2014). *Le nuvole di Picasso. Una bambina nella storia del Manicomio liberato.* Feltrinelli Editore.

[7] Bucaccio, E., Colja, K., Sermoneta, A., Turco, M. (2011). *C'era una volta la città dei matti.* Alpha Beta Verlag.

[8] Piccione, D. (2013). *Il pensiero lungo. Franco Basaglia e la Costituzione.* Alpha Beta Verlag.

[9] De Girolamo G. (1989). Italian psychiatry and reform law: a review of the international literature. *The International journal of social psychiatry, 35*(1), 21–37. https://doi.org/10.1177/002076408903500103.

[10] Cuppini, L. (2009). Il giallo del maestro «anarchico» morto durante il ricovero coatto. *Corriere della Sera, Cronache.* https://www.corriere.it/cronache/09_agosto_19/vallo_lucania_morto_trattamento_sanitario_obbligatorio_inchiesta_32ee0720-8cd2-11de-90bb-00144f02aabc.shtml.

reformed, and Ignazio Marino decided to start from those dark, forgotten places, the Forensic Psychiatric Hospitals.[11]

The inmates were often found in distressing conditions; many of the buildings housing the FPHs were derelict, overrun with rats, rain seeping in through cracks in the ceilings, no heating and lavatories that didn't bear looking at.[12] Overcrowding was rife and equipment for treatment of the disorders practically non-existent. Marino reported his findings to Giorgio Napolitano, then President of the Italian Republic, who went so far as to say that the FPHs would be inconceivable in a barely civilized country ... and were a reality that humiliated Italy before the rest of Europe ... an unspeakable horror.[13] The writing had appeared on the wall for the FPHs. They had been weighed on the scales and found lacking. They were to be closed. While undoubtedly this was a positive development from many points of view, this decision raised many problems, the same that Dr. Dell'Acqua and his colleagues were discussing that day in Trieste, starting from the question of the danger to society of these *mad criminals*, to their capacity to understand the gravity of their acts and whether these acts could be imputed to them.

In the paper mentioned earlier, Franco Rotelli expressed the opinion that "In 2012, renewing by law the legitimacy of the concept of social dangerousness linked to infirmity of mind (a concept which at this point in time is considered by legal experts and psychiatrists alike to be without any scientific or empirical grounds) and the notion of legal incompetence, which has also been strongly criticized over the last decades, implies assuming the grave responsibility of opposing the spirit and the terms of Law 180/78 that abolished the link between mental illness and social

[11] Saccomanno, M. Bosone, D. (2011). Commissione parlamentare di inchiesta sull'efficacia e l'efficienza del servizio sanitario nazionale. Relazione sulle condizioni di vita e di cura all'interno degli ospedali psichiatrici giudiziari. https://www.senato.it/documenti/repository/commissioni/servizio_sanitario16/Relazione_OOPPGG_doc_XXII-bis_4.pdf.

[12] Saccomanno, M. Bosone, D. (2011). Commissione parlamentare di inchiesta sull'efficacia e l'efficienza del servizio sanitario nazionale. Relazione sulle condizioni di vita e di cura all'interno degli ospedali psichiatrici giudiziari. https://www.senato.it/documenti/repository/commissioni/servizio_sanitario16/Relazione_OOPPGG_doc_XXII-bis_4.pdf.

[13] Napolitano, G. (2011). https://archivio.quirinale.it/discorsi-bookreader//discorsi/Viaggio_in_Italia_discorsi_interventi_Napolitano_2011_2012.html#page/46/mode/2up.

dangerousness, strenuously upholding the responsibility and the rights of every member of the community, including the right to be judged and, if guilty of the crime, to be sentenced."[14]

Franco Corleone, who was nominated by the Cabinet in 2016 as sole Commissioner for the procedures to be enforced regarding the closure of the FPHs and the completion of the REMS in certain Italian regions, commented in a convention in 2008 that he had presented a draft law under the title "Imputability of the mentally infirm person who has committed a crime and how that person is dealt with in the prison environment" in which was stated, "There are two fundamental points: (a) a mental illness shall not be considered sufficient reason to limit personal freedom if the commission of a crime has not yet been ascertained, and (b) the restriction of the liberty of a mentally infirm person having committed a crime cannot be indefinite, nor can it be temporally superior to the maximum penalty established by law for that crime. The right to be judged and the possibility of working through, processing dramatic and even tragic events must not automatically be subject to expiating the sentence in prison, i.e., in a closed institution; when there is incompatibility with detention [in prison] the possibility of serving the sentence in alternative therapeutic institutions must be taken into consideration."[15]

On my return to university in Monza, I reviewed the topics discussed in Trieste with my professor and from these discussions emerged the idea of undertaking a research project on the FPHs that could develop into a book.

While on vacation in Sicily in December 2012, I decided to visit the FPH in Barcellona Pozzo di Gotto. Dr. Dell'Acqua had provided me with a telephone number for Father Giuseppe Insana (affectionately known as *Padre Pippo*), the chaplain of the hospital and founder of the *Casa di Solidarietà e Accoglienza*, a halfway house for the inmates. I arrived in

[14] Rotelli, F., Gallio, G., Dell'Acqua, P., Del Giudice, G., Carrino, L., Novello, M. et al. (2012). *A proposito della chiusura dell'Ospedale Psichiatrico Giudiziario: le buone intenzioni di una legge pericolosa*. https://www.lavoroculturale.org/reparto-agitati-3-a-proposito-della-chiusura-dellospedale-psichiatrico-giudiziario/franco-rotelli/2012/.

[15] Corleone, F. (2008). La rimozione dell'Ospedale Psichiatrico. Speech given at the convention "La Psichiatria a 30 anni dalla Legge 180", Treviglio. https://www.fuoriluogo.it/speciali/la-rimozione-dellospedale-psichiatrico-giudiziario/.

Barcellona Pozzo di Gotto by train on December 4, 2012; while I was waiting for Padre Pippo, I was struck by a headline on the local paper, "*23-year-old youth shot dead in a barber's shop*". It was a brusque introduction to the harsh reality of the town.

Padre Pippo is a man who lives life to the full. He started his *career* as a parish priest for Santa Lucia in Barcellona Pozzo di Gotto and then became involved in Pierre Teilhard de Chardin's movement, after which he left the parish and chose to become a *worker priest*, laboring as an agricultural worker in the Sicilian countryside. During that time, he had his first encounters with the mentally infirm in the Barcellona Pozzo di Gotto FPH, who then started to spend time with him. He applied for the post of chaplain to the hospital and celebrated his first mass there on Christmas Eve 1984. "I didn't just say the mass", he confided, "I took the inmates cigarettes as well." Immediately after, in 1995, he invited some of the inmates to spend their leave in his house. Prior to that, only inmates who had enough money to pay for hotel accommodation were allowed to leave the FPH on leave.

With a group of friends from Barcellona he founded an association, the *Casa di Solidareità e Accoglienza Associazione*, which offers the inmates hospitality and helps them to find work. The Association collaborates with the Mental Health Centers. In 2000 a protocol was signed with the Department of Mental Health of Messina, the Management of the FPH and the External Relations Office of the Penitentiary with the objective of developing innovative services outside the prison walls for the FPH inmates. It was both revolutionary and successful; some of the inmates saw their security measures transformed into probation, preceding by several years the decisions of the Italian Constitutional Court[16] that definitively confirmed the possibility of assigning the mentally infirm who had committed a crime to structures other than the FPHs for treatment and reduction of their social dangerousness.

---

[16] Decisions 253/2003 and 367/2004. https://giurcost.org/decisioni/2003/0253s-03.html.

https://www.cortecostituzionale.it/actionSchedaPronuncia.do?param_ecli=ECLI:IT:COST:2004:367#:~:text=253%20del%202003%20della%20Corte%20costituzionale%20ha%20dichiarato%20illegittimo%20l,misura%20di%20sicurezza%20non%20detentiva.

When we arrived at the *Casa*, there was a welcome committee formed by a group of inmates waiting at the door. I was accosted by a large man with a black goatee and another with a form of paresis who wanted to know when I would be coming back as they had many things they wanted to tell me. Lunch was taken at a long refectory table, the food—all local produce—was blessed. Some of the guests talked and discussed vivaciously, others were absorbed in their own thoughts. The *Casa* has a list of rules to be observed: drug addicts and alcoholics are not admitted; everyone manages their own finances; medicines are placed on the table; there are no waiters, everyone does their part. Padre Pippo explained that the spirit of the *Casa* is that the Association collaborates with the inmates, helping them to help themselves. "There is a father here too", he said, "we keep in touch with the families, the inmates have the possibility of going home and of calling home. Inside the FPH there are no rules, here we have small rules for cohabitation: everyone is treated as a person. And the bread and cakes come from the best bakery in Barcellona!".

In the afternoon Padre Pippo accompanied me to the FPH and introduced me to the Director, Dr. Nunziante Rosania, a medical doctor and criminologist, who was well disposed to answering my questions regarding the FPH and the investigation launched by the Commission headed by Senator Marino. He had been responsible for the FPH since 1997 and was particularly proud of the fact that in his first ten years the use of antipsychotic drugs had been considerably reduced, so improving the inmates' quality of life.

"There is no reason that these individuals should not live outside the prison. In my view, they are people who are distressed. The walls, the restrictions, come later. The question, where should we put them? That comes later. Mental illness is a classification. On this point, I do not agree with the idea that mental illness is simply a product of society. Mental illness requires a psychiatric clinic, awareness and scientific rigor. My view of mental illness is that it has a genetic origin that interpenetrates with the environmental component, which is much more important. The FPH is an institution that doesn't take the individual into consideration." Having said this, he stared me in the eye and said, "Well, what kind of psychiatrist do you want to be? One who works with the patients, or one who sits behind a desk?".

Ignazio Marino visited Barcellona Pozzo di Gotto for the first time in June 2010 (the Director was not present that day) and returned in December, after visiting the other five FPHs. According to Dr. Rosania, "They filmed the worst situations, the ones that were guaranteed to scandalize. They even filmed that famous iron bed, the one with the hole. We have always used a restraint bed in the isolation cell for pantoclastic crises. For each case, we write up a number of reports. One for the agent, one for the ward doctor, one for the highest-ranking prison officer, one for the psychiatrist who ordered the restraint to control the crisis (three hours maximum), the ward commander, the director who authorizes the restraint. There are two reports, one medical and one psychiatric. When I arrived in 1997 there were 27 restraint beds, now there is only one. The person they filmed tied to the bed was Mr. C, nicknamed the Cardinal because he had a mole shaped like cardinal's hat, like Gorbachev. In the report they said the mole was a bruise caused by the restraint. In May 2012 we had a visit from the European Committee for the Prevention of Torture comprised of eight experts: psychiatrists, prison directors, with French/Italian interpreters. They arrived at 8 am on May 15 and left at 8 pm on May 16. They visited everything. At the end of their visit, we had a debriefing session and this is what they said, 'We can't understand why Marino reached the conclusions he did. You are doing very high standard work with the human and professional resources that are available to you. Our congratulations to you, but not to the Italian State that leaves you to work in these very difficult conditions.' Twenty days later I got a letter of praise from the Minister of Justice. It makes you wonder."

On my return, I contacted Caterina Clerici, a journalist-photographer,[17] as I hoped to add some visual documentation along the lines of the book by Valeria P. Babini, *Liberi tutti. Manicomi e psichiatri in Italia.*[18] I had

[17] Caterina Clerici is an Italian freelance journalist, currently based in New York. She focuses on international development and human rights, as well as migration and integration issues. Her work has appeared on The Guardian, Al Jazeera English, La Stampa, Repubblica, Libération, The Independent, Slate and TIME, where she also works as a photo editor. Caterina holds a bachelor's degree in Politics and Development Studies from the School of Oriental and African Studies in London, and a master's degree from Columbia University's Graduate Journalism School.

[18] Babini, V.P. (2009). *Liberi tutti. Manicomi e psichiatri in Italia.* Il Mulino.

seen an exhibition of Caterina's work and had been very impressed by her photographs of Liberian men, women and children and how she had caught the intensity of their expressions; I could imagine how she would capture the inmates of the FPHs on film. In the months after my return I had also submitted the project for approval to the University of Milano-Bicocca and to the Penitentiary Administration Department in Rome. The project was approved and I was granted access to all six FPHs.

I went back to Barcellona Pozzo di Gotto in February 2013 to see how I could develop the project. I stayed in the *Casa* and discussed the best way to proceed with Padre Pippo and his guests. The idea was to interview the inmates to listen to their life stories, understand their language, their imagery, their experiences before and after acquittal and how they spend their days in the FPH. While I was there, one of the FPH wards was being closed; Padre Pippo provided me with the press reports and the laws and sentences regarding this historical happening. The structure had been seized by order of Senator Marino on December 19, 2012; the inmates were to have been transferred within thirty days, subsequently extended to February 12 and then to March 31, 2013. The order was never executed.

In September 2013, I left for Barcellona Pozzo di Gotto with Caterina. We visited Reggio Emilia in February 2014, followed by Castiglione delle Stiviere, Aversa, Naples and in the September of that year, Montelupo Fiorentino, the last visit. 2014 was a year of intense debate on the FPHs and the decision to postpone the date of the closures to March 31, 2015. It was the second extension.

I was extremely fortunate to have witnessed the end of this institution from the inside, to have been able to experience at first hand the dynamics and organization of a controversial reality often under attack from various quarters, to collect impressions from the inmates before their transfer to the Residences for the Execution of Security Measures (the REMS); it was an unforgettable experience from both the human and the professional standpoints.

I had conversations with many of the inmates; some were brief, not even thirty minutes in length, while others extended for over an hour, but all were intense, revealing complex and transversal cross-sections of society. I used a list of standard questions, touching on the following themes:

the type of crime and consequent sentence; a description of their experiences in prison and FPH; the origin and their awareness of their mental illness; what, in their view, is a mental illness; what, in their view, is social dangerousness; what therapy are they taking; their typical day in the FPH; their expectations and prospects for the future. All the inmates gave their written consent to the interviews and their subsequent publication. The Directors of Reggio Emilia, Barcellona Pozzo di Gotto and Montelupo Fiorentino, respectively Drs. Paolo Madonna, Nunziante Rosania and Antonella Tuoni, consented to the interviews and the photographic reportage as agreed with Dr. Calogero R. Piscitello, General Director of the Penitentiary Administration Department.

When I started work on this project in 2013, there was a great deal of feeling and discussion about the FPHs following the revelations of the Parliamentary Commission of Inquiry. It was important to document this last act of a long era of Italian psychiatry, Caterina with her camera and me with the documentation gathered from the inmates and the staff. The media was very active and was exerting pressure on the political decisions that were delaying the closure of the FPHs. Caterina made her own contribution to clarifying the situation, writing articles and providing photographic documentation for the Italian daily La Stampa.[19, 20]

The interviews with the inmates revealed a perspective of the FPH that was far more informative than the reports on the press. Their accounts did not contain any talk of scandalous happenings, they were stories of personal drama, episodes of violence and murder that had altered social equilibrium. Illness combined with disorders that had never been treated, with degradation of the environment, drug abuse and alcoholism. There were stories of odysseys from one prison to another, from a hospital to a rehab community, finishing up in an FPH. I had a wealth of material, the question was, what to do with it? I toyed with the idea of a collection of

[19] Clerici, C. (2014). Tra crimine e follia. https://www.lastampa.it/torino/2014/06/03/news/tra-crimine-e-follia-1.35740122/; Clerici, C. (2015). Viaggio negli Ospedali Psichiatrici Giudiziari. https://www.lastampa.it/cronaca/2015/03/29/fotogalleria/viaggio-negli-ospedali-psichiatrici-giudiziari-1.35289117.

[20] Russo, P., Clerici, C. (photographs). (2015). La chiusura degli OPG spaventa medici e pm: "Rischi per la sicurezza". https://www.lastampa.it/cronaca/2015/03/29/news/la-chiusura-degli-opg-spaventa-medici-e-pm-rischi-per-la-sicurezza-1.35288865.

stories, a sociological snapshot of *criminal madmen* to lower the curtain on the FPHs. It would have been a page in the history of Italian psychiatry, but it would refer only to the past and most likely would be eclipsed by the long-awaited law decreeing the closure. With Caterina, I decided to use some of the material immediately for journalistic purposes, and with the remainder, write a book starting from the stories of the inmates, and enriched with reflections on their disorders, their distress, and the task of integrating these inmates, in all their complexity, in the new therapeutic centers. It would be a clinical and psychiatric text, without neglecting the protagonists themselves and their experiences. I started work on the book after the opening of the REMS, while concluding the first stage of my psychiatric studies.

The first task was to select the material to be used, and I decided on the interviews obtained in Reggio Emilia, Barcellona Pozzo di Gotto and Montelupo Fiorentino. This choice was dictated not by the space available, but by the suitability of the material for the structure of the book, the testimony of the inmates followed by an essay. Each story was obviously unique, giving rise to many questions regarding the treatments, the work of the psychiatrists and health workers.

The book is structured in three sections, one for each FPH, preceded by an introduction including a history of the building, and a comment on my experiences there. The introduction to Reggio Emilia recounts the working climate and meetings I had with the staff, that to Barcellona Pozzo di Gotto a comment on the life in the *Casa della Solidarietà e Accoglienza*, while the introduction to Montelupo Fiorentino contains an interview with Dr. Franco Scarpa, the director in that period, and his collaborators, Antonella Lettieri, psychologist and Maria Rosaria Capone and Luca Bigalli, psychiatrists. Each section contains six interviews, in the language used by the inmates themselves which at times may appear confused, at others extremely lucid, so as to pick up the message underlying the actual words, frequently communicated with details, nuances, expressions, neologisms. For each FPH I have selected three cases for an in-depth analysis to throw light on the inmate's account, inserting it into a psychopathological framework, with notes on the therapy, treatment options and open questions.

Why did I decide to write about the FPHs and in these terms? For many years these institutions were on the fringe of society, at best forgotten but mainly ignored. It wasn't until the middle of the twentieth century that adverse reports began to appear, enquiries were made and essays written, mainly in the wake of Franco Basaglia's new vision of psychiatry. There were several journalistic investigations into the degradation of certain structures and the living conditions. There was much talk about reforms but nothing happened until after Senator Marino's Parliamentary Commission. Reviewing the available documentation, it seemed to me that a critical factor was missing, nowhere could I find a profile of the inmates of the FPH. I felt it was important to take the extraordinary opportunity of visiting these structures in their final days to fill this lacuna, and to tell the stories of the inmates who would soon be transferred to new structures, structures without bars at the windows and locks on the doors, designed to rehabilitate people who have committed a crime while affected by psychic pathologies.

This book is intended as a case study: much can be learnt from these stories of life in the FPHs regarding the precautions to be taken to avoid repeating the mistakes of the past and to adopt practices that respect the individual and are more flexible in searching for rehabilitation methods. These stories are an invitation to adopt best practices that are in the process of being adopted here and at international level.

It was never easy crossing the threshold of an FPH. Imposing doors opened silently and closed behind us immediately. There were moments of anxiety when we met the prison guard. Sometimes they would tell us how to reach our destination and send us on our way alone, sometimes they accompanied us. The day was full of surprises and the unexpected: who would we be talking to? How would they react to the interview? Where would the story take us? These were stories of another world, a parallel world filled with drama, suffering, violence, pilgrimages from prisons to hospitals, stories of therapies tried and therapies rejected, of restraints and abandon, of visions and persecution manias, of real memories and wild imagination. Everything had a strange aura, from the gardens to the corridors, the entrance halls to the individual cells filled with objects that had no connection to the occupant, an unfamiliar place that would never become familiar. We felt we were being watched: we were outsiders, foreigners. When we met the gaze of an inmate, we caught a fleeting glimpse of a drama unfolding, sometimes perceptible by the lines traced on the face, the expression, the eyes, at other times unfathomable without the comments of the doctors and health workers accompanying us. The interviews, so different one from another, opened ancient wounds and revealed family scenarios, sometimes fraught with misery, sometimes a love story defeated by the illness. Even when the story was rich in detail, we had the impression that we had only scratched the surface of the humanity before us. We saw much, but we glimpsed so much more. So much was hidden.

Each story offers a cross-section of life and illness, of behavior and delirium, life, suffering without end. Each story remains open and at every new reading other questions come to mind, that bring with them new imagery and hypotheses. There is always something different to be glimpsed. The person suffering from a psychic disorder communicates a sense of vagueness, which on the one hand expresses the nature of the illness, on the other their unpredictable response to the therapy. Even those patients who have not committed any crime, who follow their therapy religiously and tell their doctor everything, still have an area of the mind that remains unfathomable, concealed by the illness, where you can formulate hypotheses, but can go no further with any certainty. Indeed, the inhabitants of the world of mental illness are to a great extent invisible, and only those of us who have a relative or friend who suffers from a psychic disorder and those who work in the sector can have an idea of the anguish involved.

There is a story that epitomizes *this seeing beyond the physical* that was described in a book by Daniele Mencarelli, *La casa degli sguardi*. He tells of a nun in the children's hospital in Rome who came across a child with a terribly deformed head and laid her cheek against their's. His main character muses, "I saw something familiar and at the same time foreign, like a strange rite from a far off country, but I can't seem to find the instruments to translate it into my language." What did the nun see in the little patient? Everyone looks at the patients in the ward, but some people see more than others, like the nun who smiled at the child and said to him, "You are your mother and father's *darling*, aren't you?".

The protagonists of this book are "criminal madmen" or "mad criminals", at the farthest extreme of the spectrum of mental disorder; the mystery is whether it was this disorder that led them to commit their crime, or whether the illness arrived later, during confinement. They have one thing in common: living inside the FPH, they are ghosts for those who live on the outside. They exist but are not visible, they are lost to those who live outside the walls of those very institutions where many of them have spent most of their lives, concealed from the eyes of the world. People who are considered a danger to society are kept hidden, segregated in impenetrable buildings, and so acquire a veil of mystery.[21] But the people in this book came forward to tell their story and so have become visible through their testimony, shedding a little of that mystery that surrounds psychic disorders and offering a glimpse of their world. As Lorenzo Calvi said, "the feelers of the phenomenologist start to vibrate when s/he receives the gift of vision, that is, when, in the world of objects, one is suffused with splendor and so stands out from the others, appearing as a glimpse".[22] A glimpse that we hope can arouse curiosity to see more, to understand, to empathize.

[21] Foucault, M. (2009). *History of Madness*. Routledge.

[22] Calvi, L. (2005). *Il tempo dell'altro significato*. Mimesis. ISBN: 9788884833006.

2

About Psychiatry

Mental Illness[1]

Mental illness is a mystery. It is a condition affecting a person's ontological dimension[2] that can also have negative effects on their body. It cannot be fully explained by biological mechanisms, although progress is being made in that direction, as in the study of genetics and the neuroimaging techniques that investigate the cerebral areas involved in certain disorders. Maybe the best way to define mental illness in this context is to consider the mentally ill, taking into account my ten years of experience working in this field. The mentally ill, or psychiatric patient (a term I prefer not to use, as it is too narrow as a definition, linking the identity of the person to the discipline and consequently to the power this discipline can exert on the patient), is a person whose mind, or psyche, is affected, distorted even, by a disorder. Here we could open a debate as to what

[1] The term 'mental illness' covers a vast number of mental illnesses or disorders with different etiopathogenesis, clinical courses, and treatments. Here the term is used in the singular form in order to focus on the totality of the problem, with no intention of ignoring the importance of the development of the various disorders. This was the approach adopted during the interviews with the individual patients, who were asked for their thoughts on mental illness.

[2] Binswanger, L. (1992). *Der Mensch in der Psychiatrie.* Pfullingen.

J. Santambrogio, *Stories from Italian Forensic Psychiatric Hospitals*,
https://doi.org/10.1007/978-3-031-61129-2_2

exactly is meant by "mind" and "psyche" and their relation to the brain, which however is not usually included in definitions of this typology of patient and illness, even though it is the somatic base in which psychic processes take place.[3] In recent years neuroscience has made enormous progress, arriving at the concept of embodied mind[4, 5] and so avoiding the Cartesian mind/body dichotomy.[6] It has been known for some time that all mental activity produces functional modifications of the brain, and the entire body.[7] According to biological psychiatry, all mental disorders can and must be seen as illnesses of the brain, or brain disorders; the supporters of this theory have developed a research network complementary to the Diagnostic and Statistical Manual to study mental health and illnesses according to biological parameters, from genetics to cerebral circuits, from behavior to self-reports (Research Domain Criteria, R-DoC).[8] However, at the time of writing, there has not yet been an epistemological change in the nature of psychiatry.

Unlike the brain, mind and psyche conjure up images of volatile, evanescent, ephemeral entities; however, notwithstanding this intangibility they are decisive in determining the thoughts and emotions that also guide the body. Disorders of the mind, therefore, are disorders that affect thoughts (thoughts in the sense of psychic function), sense perception, mood, and affectivity extending to external aspects such as appearance, the ability to mimic, expressions. Sometimes they appear suddenly, out of the blue, but more often they develop in phases as in schizophrenia,[9] in which the basic symptoms, i.e., the constellation of subjective symptoms

[3] Castellano, F., Carrà, G., Santambrogio, J., Clerici, M. (2014). Comportamento emozionale patologico. In Papagno, C., Gallace, A., (eds.) *Psicobiologia del comportamento normale e patologico.*

[4] Edelman, G. M. (2006). *Second Nature.* Yale University Press.

[5] Kandel, E. R. (2005). *Psychiatry, psychoanalysis, and the new biology of mind.* American Psychiatric Publishing, Inc.

[6] Damasio, A. (2005). *Descartes' Error.* Penguin.

[7] Carta, I., Santambrogio, J. (2010). Mente-Cervello: enigma scientifico o mistero? In Cornaggia, C.M., Clerici, M., Zappa, L.E. (eds.). La sindrome di Lazzaro, morte della follia e psichiatria pubblica. 8. Libreria al Segno.

[8] Clark, L. A., Cuthbert, B., Lewis-Fernández, R., Narrow, W. E., & Reed, G. M. (2017). Three approaches to understanding and classifying mental disorder: *ICD-11*, *DSM-5*, and the National Institute of Mental Health's Research Domain Criteria (RDoC). *Psychological Science in the Public Interest, 18*(2), 72–145. https://doi.org/10.1177/1529100617727266

[9] Stangellini, G. (1992). *Verso la schizofrenia, la teoria dei sintomi base.* Idelson Liviana.

of which the person becomes aware, evolve into the delusional mood phase (*wahnstimmung*) in which the affective range becomes increasingly persecutory in nature, culminating in the onset of psychosis with delirium (the *epiphany of delirium*) and, in some cases, body image disturbance.[10, 11] OCD (Obsessive-compulsive disorder) or phobias, which fall under the category of neurosis, can also develop in a similarly insidious manner.[12] Bipolarism is another example of a mental disorder that is difficult to diagnose in the early stages; it is hereditary, but onset is triggered by the interaction of genes and the environment. Frequently, the person themselves and their relations do not understand the significance and importance of the symptoms of this disorder, which may also manifest as hypomanic or manic episodes.[13] Research in psychoeducation has contributed to providing assistance to families for the treatment of this disorder.[14]

The onset of a mental disorder frequently involves the members of the person's family; it can be compared to an earthquake, shaking the very foundations of family life. In the beginning, the members of the family may be gripped with anxiety by their relative's strange and unpredictable behavior. Some experience feelings of guilt, others are ashamed and attempt to isolate and hide the person with the mental disorder because they reflect a situation of distress within the family. Others again simply deny the evidence and continue their life as normal, pretending that nothing untoward is happening. These cases frequently culminate in a tragic outcome as the disorder, left untreated, becomes increasingly serious. The situation may however reach the point when one or more members of the family accept that there is something wrong and take steps to find a solution.

---

[10] Ballerini, A., Rossi, Monti, M. (2011). *La Vergogna e il delirio, un modello delle sindromi paranoidee.* Giovanni Fioriti Editore.

[11] Ballerini, A., Di Petta, G. (2015). *Oltre e di là del mondo: l'essenza della schizophrenia. Fenomenologia e Psicopatologia.* Giovanni Fioriti Editore.

[12] Calvi, L. (2005). *Il tempo dell'altro significato. Esercizi fenomenologici d'uno psichiatra.* Mimesis.

[13] Vieta, E., Berk, M., Schulze, T. G., Carvalho, A. F., Suppes, T., Calabrese, J. R., Gao, K., Miskowiak, K. W., & Grande, I. (2018). Bipolar disorders. *Nature Reviews Disease Primers*, 4(1). https://doi.org/10.1038/nrdp.2018.8

[14] Colom, F., & Vieta, E. (2006). *Psychoeducation Manual for Bipolar Disorder.* Cambridge University Press.

This is where reconstruction, so fundamental for treatment, must start. In the family. After all, who knows the patient better than a parent or a close relative? They can generally help in those crucial moments in life, for example, a mental breakdown. A kind word, some sound advice, a sign of empathy, can be decisive in supporting a person in mental distress. Of course, as Franco Basaglia said, "Everything has its double".[15] When family members are tormented by anxiety, frustrated by strange behavior, and beset by a sense of guilt, it is unlikely they will be able to act in a positive manner towards the patient. These forms of distress are contagious and soon spread. Once the family has come to terms with the fact that the problem is not of a nature to be treated with the usual domestic remedies, help and advice about what should be done is sought outside the immediate family circle. Friends and relatives are consulted; in some cases, help will be asked from the local priest. Sooner or later, however, a decision must made and the family will turn to the family doctor, or a Mental Health Service Centre or a psychiatrist. Frequently, this decision will be postponed for as long as possible (and in some cases even longer) due to a negative perception of psychiatry and psychiatrists. When it is no longer possible to put off action, the next question is whom to consult? Which branch of psychiatry?[16]

Who, then, is the psychiatrist? What does professionalism and "being professional" mean for a psychiatrist? According to the American psychiatrist Glen Gabbard and his colleagues (Gabbard et al., 2012), "Cultural sensitivity is at the heart of the psychiatrist's professional identity. Psychiatrists attempt to understand patients in their biopsychosocial context, honoring the many factors that shape an individual's life. One cannot completely transcend the influence of one's own culture. Psychiatrists, by the very nature of their practice, are prone to think about the uniqueness of each individual and, unlike other physicians, tend to value the multiplicity and complexity of each individual. Patients are not regarded reductionistically and simplistically as a

[15] Basaglia, F. (1985). What Is Psychiatry? *International Journal of Mental Health*, 14(1), 42–51. https://doi.org/10.1080/00207411.1985.11448987

[16] Santambrogio, J., Clerici, M. (2012). Pazienti, psichiatrici e famiglia. Il contributo dei Servizi pubblici. *Famiglia Oggi,* 3, 14–15.

disease process. A psychiatric disorder occurs in a person (Gabbard 2005), a whole, unique person in a rich and multifaceted context."[17]

The psychiatrist is always faced with a clinically complex person, complex also in their relationships. According to Gabbard, the level of ethics and rigor that must accompany psychiatrists in their venture, as it leads to a knowledge of human fragility and greatness, must exceed that required even from the family doctor. Whoever works in the field of psychiatry is aware of the delicacy of the doctor-patient relationship. This is a profession that requires constant study, research, and practice in the field under the supervision of experienced colleagues, the psychiatrist who simply uses intuition is placing both him/herself and the patient at risk.

Returning to the definition of mental illness, it must be added that in the acute phase the disorder can seriously condition the behavior of the person, their understanding of their actions and the consequences thereof (the ability to comprehend) or, if their faculty of comprehension remains intact, their capacity to control their actions may be damaged, and they will perform an action even though they realize it will have negative consequences. In extreme czases both these faculties are compromised, and the person is considered to be of unsound mind. A psychotic in a phase of pathopsychological deficit could commit an act of violence if, for example, he is in a blind alley and is convinced he is being followed by persons with hostile intent. A man who has been abandoned by his companion, wounded in his pride and unable to process what has happened, could find himself unable to resist the temptation to stalk the woman, threaten her and in an escalation of rage, pass from psychological to physical violence. If, in these two hypothetical cases, the protagonists do in fact commit an act of violence, they will (in all probability) be apprehended by the appropriate authorities and a psychiatric assessment will be requested. In this case, the expert who conducts the assessment has the task of ascertaining whether the person was of unsound mind at the time they committed the violence, whether they constitute a danger to others and to themselves, their fitness to plead, and where they should be sent.

[17] Gabbard, G.O., Roberts, L.W., Crisp-Han, H., Ball, V., Hobday, G., & Rachal, F. (2012). *Professionalism in Psychiatry*. American Psychiatric Pub.

The magistrate, having heard the evidence and perused the psychiatric assessment, may decide to acquit the person, establishing that they are not guilty in the classical sense of the term, because they were of unsound mind. This means that the person will not be sent to prison to serve a sentence but will be placed in a secure hospital setting (originally the FPH, now the REMS) where he will receive treatment, but at the same time, being held under a security measure, he will have his liberty restricted and will be separated from society to avoid the risk of a repetition of his crime.

The Condition of the Mentally Infirm in Italy

Forty years have passed since the Basaglia Law (1978) came into force, establishing the closure of the mental asylums, and during this period assistance to the mentally infirm in Italy has changed radically. Those provincial institutions, the mental asylums, are no more. These structures that were dedicated to the treatment and restraint of mental illnesses and intended to hide people considered to be a scandal, and often, dangerous, from the public view, exist no longer. Today, assistance for people with mental disorders is based on a territorial system, revolving around the Mental Health Centers, Psychosocial Centers or Centers for Mental Hygiene. They provide regular psychiatric visits, nursing support, and social support for patients who are suffering from an insidious and often long-term illness that impairs their health, relationships, work, personal independence, even their future.

The objective of these centers is to provide treatment and services to the mentally infirm on their home ground, in order to promote their integration into society and maintain their significant relationships; this, however, is not as easy as it might sound as they have to manage large numbers of patients and complex situations. Grave cases of psychopathology often involve social and even legal problems, so the treatment must shift to the social control that Basaglia's reforms intended to exclude from the competences of psychiatry. Another problem is the high staff turnover, psychiatrists first and foremost. This is particularly difficult for the patients, who must tell their story again from the start each time a new doctor is assigned to them. The doctors themselves tend to see their position as temporary and so, rather than dedicating time to listening to the patient and understanding the case history fully, they pass directly to a diagnosis and therapy.[18]

Acute cases are referred to the Psychiatric Services for Diagnosis and Treatment, which are wards with a maximum of 15 beds, reserved for the purpose in the general hospitals.

A study conducted by Prof. Giovanni de Girolamo and colleagues and published in 2007[19] found that in Italy at that time there were 4,113 beds in public structures for acute cases, an average of 0.78 beds for ten thousand inhabitants, which is approximately 20% less than the national standard. There were also 4,862 beds in 54 private clinics making a total of 8,975 beds in Italy (excluding Sicily) for short term, acute cases. By 2014, the situation had improved slightly to 10.95 beds per one hundred thousand inhabitants as reported by Corrado Barbui and his colleagues in their article published in 2018.[20]

Hospitalization in these wards can be prescribed following a check-up by territorial psychiatrists, but in many cases it is the patients themselves, accompanied by a family member, who go to the hospital A & E or call emergency services and request admittance. The psychiatrist on call in the hospital makes an initial assessment in the A & E to decide whether the patient's condition is severe enough to merit admittance to the ward. These assessments are frequently carried out under difficult circumstances: on the one hand, the condition of the patient (for example, a psychotic disorder with hallucinations, suicidal intent, serious depression) and on the other, the possibility of substance abuse which can act as a catalyst on the psychic disorder and may culminate in violent behavior.

---

[18] Tibaldi, G. (2018). Il contributo dei servizi ai processi di cronicizzazione. Quali ombre del manicomio gravano ancora sulle pratiche della "nostra" psichiatria di comunità? *Rivista Sperimentale Di Freniatria*, *3*, 9–17. https://doi.org/10.3280/rsf2018-003002

[19] De Girolamo, G., Barbato, A., Bracco, R., Gaddini, A., Miglio, R., Morosini, P., Norcio, B., Picardi, A., Rossi, E., Rucci, P., Santone, G., Dell'Acqua, G., & PROGRES-Acute group (2007). Characteristics and activities of acute psychiatric in-patient facilities: national survey in Italy. *The British journal of psychiatry: the journal of mental science*, *191*, 170–177. https://doi.org/10.1192/bjp.bp.105.020636.

[20] Barbui, C., Papola, D., & Saraceno, B. (2018). Forty years without mental hospitals in Italy. *International Journal of Mental Health Systems*, *12*(1). https://doi.org/10.1186/s13033-018-0223-1.

When this happens, the A & E staff assist the psychiatrist in restraining the patient (to avoid causing injury to themselves and to other people present) and injecting a sedative. In cases of severe psychopathologies that require urgent treatment where the patient does not acknowledge the problem and refuses the treatment, the doctor can order a Compulsory Sanitary Treatment (TSO in Italian). This must be validated by another doctor and authorized by the mayor; it has a duration of seven days (renewable). The Compulsory Sanitary Treatment is regulated by article 34 of Law 833/78 and it is interesting to note how the number of admissions following orders of this type has decreased over the years: from 50% in 1975 (three years prior to Law 833) to 25.84% in 1978 (over 20,000 admissions), to 18.10% in 1985, 11.60% in 1995, 4.15% in 2005 and 4.71% in 2015 (less than 9,000 admissions).[21] This could be interpreted as a gradual improvement in the assistance provided to the mentally infirm, the transition from a custodial format (the asylums) to a more humane form of treatment. The suicide rate among psychiatric patients since 1978 has remained stable in spite of the decrease in beds available. In 1978, 7.1 suicides were recorded per 100,000 inhabitants, 8.8 in 1985, 5.6 in 2006 and 6.3 in 2012. There does not seem to be a relation between the decrease in the number of beds available for psychiatric patients since 1978, and the numbers of Compulsory Sanitary Treatment and suicides.[22]

The Psychiatric Services for Diagnosis and Treatment undoubtedly provide a useful service to the mentally infirm, however they sometimes become a kind of "sorting house", simply directing the patients to other solutions, e.g., treatment at home, rehabilitation communities, other institutions. It is the staff that makes the difference; the warmer the welcome, and the more attentive the listener to the patient's problems, the more likely it is that the patient will feel protected and reassured, and will be collaborative in following the prescribed course of treatment, full of hope for a change in their condition.[23] Unfortunately, what often happens

---

[21] Data from the National Research Institute—ISTAT.

[22] Barbui, C., Papola, D., & Saraceno, B. (2018). Forty years without mental hospitals in Italy. *International Journal of Mental Health Systems, 12*(1). https://doi.org/10.1186/s13033-018-0223-1.

[23] Ducci, G. (2010). *Buone pratiche in SPDC. La costruzione di linee guida nei SPDC del Lazio*. Alpes.

is that due to the overwhelming number of requests for beds, the doctors have very little time to spend with the individual patients, the objective being to cure the patients as quickly as possible and free up beds, while the risk is that despite all good intentions, the patient will have a relapse. This phenomenon is known as "revolving doors". Another problem is the variety of typologies these centers have to deal with on a daily basis, such as inmates from prisons sent for assessment of acute disorders, mentally ill patients who have committed a crime and are still subject to a security measure, waiting to be sent to a REMS,[24] potentially violent patients with a double diagnosis (mental disorder and substance abuse), cognitively retarded patients with behavioural anomalies, the homeless who wander into an A & E and are assigned to a psychiatrist, immigrants with and without permits but with psychopathologies that are difficult to understand. Then there is the problem of restraint, the use of which is inevitable under certain conditions and may well be applied with roughness by the personnel; the patient may see this as a limitation to his personal freedom and dignity, which undermines the relationship with the psychiatrist responsible for his/her treatment.

This brief review of the treatment opportunities available to the mentally ill would not be complete without a mention of the Psychiatric Residences. Barbui and colleagues reported that in 2014 the rate of admission to Psychiatric Residences was 46.41 per 100,000 inhabitants.[25] The PROGRES (Residence project),[26] published in 2002, studied the situation of these residences in Italy (public, private non-profit, private). As of May 31, 2000, there were 1370 Residences (with at least 4 beds) with an average of 12.5 beds, i.e., 2.98 residential beds per 10,000 inhabitants. However, the availability from region to region varied greatly. The number

[24] A separate chapter will be dedicated to the REMS (residences for the execution of security measures), the structures designed for the accommodation and care of mentally ill offenders following the closure of the FPH (when the responsibility for these persons transferred from the Ministry of Justice to the Ministry of Health), the objective being to promote rehabilitation and reintegration into society.

[25] Barbui, C., Papola, D., & Saraceno, B. (2018). Forty years without mental hospitals in Italy. *International Journal of Mental Health Systems*, *12*(1). https://doi.org/10.1186/s13033-018-0223-1.

[26] de Girolamo, G., Picardi, A., Micciolo, R., Falloon, I., Fioritti, A., Morosini, P. for the Italian PROGRES study group (2002). Residential care in Italy: a national survey of non-hospital facilities. *British Journal of Psychiatry*, 181, 220–225.

of patients present in the Residences was 15,943, an average of 11.6 per residence. The patient turnover was recorded as being low. In 1999, over one third of the residences had not discharged anyone, while another third had discharged only 1 or 2 patients. Consequently, there were very few new admissions. The variables associated with the low turnover were the advanced age of the patients, a high number of residents, the presence of residents from the FPH, and staff not being present round the clock.

The question that automatically springs to mind is whether these Residences are rehabilitation centers where the patients are prepared for reintegration into the community or whether they simply offer long-term accommodation. The faces of many of the patients in these Residences are marked with the unmistakable signs of a long-term illness, which has alienated them from their homes, their work, their relationships, leading to yet another question: what is chronicity in psychiatry?

The REMS and the Patients from the FPH

As of March 31, 2015, which was the date established by Law 81/2014, there were no more admissions to the FPH, with the exception of Castiglione delle Stiviere for a limited period. When the last patient left the Barcellona Pozzo di Gotto FPH in March 2017, Italy became the first country in the world to close its Forensic Psychiatric Hospitals.[27] The psychiatric patients from these institutions who had committed crimes and had been acquitted as being unfit to stand trial were sent to the Residences for the Execution of Security Measures (REMS), institutions managed exclusively by National Health Service staff. These Residences focus on treating patients with programs designed to suit their individual needs with a view to their return to the community. At the time of the closures of the FPH there were 30 such structures, distributed over the national territory, with a total capacity for 624 patients, compared to the 1,015 patients who had been living in the FPH in the years prior to the closure. Indeed, there were long waiting lists (235 in February 2015),

[27] Di Lorito, C., Castelletti, L., Lega, I., Gualco, B., Scarpa, F., & Völlm, B. (2017). The closing of forensic psychiatric hospitals in Italy: Determinants, current status and future perspectives. A scoping review. *International journal of law and psychiatry*, *55*, 54–63. https://doi.org/10.1016/j.ijlp.2017.10.004.

with the patients waiting in prison (where psychiatric treatment was no longer available), in rehab centers managed by the Department of Mental Health, or at home, depending on the gravity of their crimes.[28] This situation gave rise to a number of concerns: how were the prison staff supposed to cope with these individuals, without any specific training? Would the rehab centers be adequately staffed to deal with such cases? How would families cope? How could security be guaranteed?

A study was conducted from June 2017 to June 2019 on 28 REMS for a total of 730 patients of whom 80 were women. The report, published in 2019, stated that the most common diagnosis was schizophrenia (33%), followed by personality disorders (32%) and disorders linked to substance abuse (21.4%). The crimes committed by the patients were recorded as murder/attempted murder (26%), grievous bodily harm, molesting (24%), domestic violence (19%), crimes against property (12%), assaulting a police officer (7%), stalking (7%), sex crimes (4%). 39% of the patients were held by a provisional measure, which is indicative of a lengthy lapse of time between the crime and the definitive sentence, and underlines the necessity of creating intermediate forensic psychiatric structures to accommodate and provide treatment for these individuals who undoubtedly represent a risk to society.[29]

The REMS and related issues are dealt with in greater depth in Chap. 5.

Open Questions

1. *Creativity as treatment and an antidote against institutionalization*

From time immemorial, poetry, art, music, theatre are all creative means of expression. An artist has the capacity to express profound sentiments in an alternative language, sentiments that are perceived by

[28] Di Lorito, C., Castelletti, L., Lega, I., Gualco, B., Scarpa, F., & Völlm, B. (2017). The closing of forensic psychiatric hospitals in Italy: Determinants, current status and future perspectives. A scoping review. *International journal of law and psychiatry, 55*, 54–63. https://doi.org/10.1016/j.ijlp.2017.10.004.

[29] Catanesi, R., Mandarelli, G., Ferracuti, S., Valerio, A., & Carabellese, F. (2019). The new Italian Residential Forensic Psychiatric System (REMS). A one-year population study. *Italian Journal Of Criminology, 13*, 7–23. https://doi.org/10.7347/ric-ns2019-p07.

intuition and sensitivity before they are processed rationally; they have the ability of morphing into another personality… they transform. After the creative act, what was there before is no longer there; it has transformed into something different, something new. And the artists, in creating, have transformed themselves by offering this contribution to the world, they have revealed something of their inner being, they have expressed a judgement on life and the environment, thus continuously renewing themselves.

The psychiatric patient is first and foremost a person with immense resources for the psychiatrist examining them in the hope of finding a diagnosis. Creativity is one of these resources, permitting the patient to find alternative channels of communication that, at least for a certain length of time, keep their obsessive, maniacal and delirious thoughts at bay. *Fausto,* the first person we spoke to in Reggio Emilia, found in poetry a lifeline that helped him resist being, turned into a chronic patient by the psychiatric institution. In his poetry he writes about the FPH, allowing his feelings to emerge, but he also writes about his relationship with God, expresses his thoughts about liberty, the strength needed to recover after a relapse. His poetry is not only inspired by the illness as such, but also and mostly by suffering, fueled by fragility and kindness. *Giancarlo* in Barcellona Pozzo di Gotto, uses the medium of a video-poem to protest about the power that psychiatry exerts over the patients. *Davide* in Reggio Emilia found a reason for living in his guitar. These cases, and there were others, surely show that investing resources in artistic activities for rehabilitation is well worth while.

2. *The patient/psychiatrist relationship.*

For a person with a mental disorder, the first meeting with the psychiatrist leaves an indelible mark. During that meeting they exchange glances and experiences, creating a relationship that would be difficult to repeat with another person under different circumstances. If the psychiatrist is well disposed to listen to the patient, then what he hears may strike an unexpected chord, recall similar nuances in his own life experience. *Fausto* stated that "the psychiatrist who understands and then adds something of his own, creates dialogue and trust together". Together they create a relationship on which to base the patient's treatment that assists with selecting the correct pharmacological cure, which although extremely important is not the be all and end all; the relationship must also help the patient recover from relapses. *Fausto* had a point of view on this aspect also, "the world of psychiatry violates you mentally, I mean when you reveal your innermost thoughts, tell everything about you, if the psychiatrist to whom you are talking hasn't had the right training, it can be a very violent experience. A medical history recorded simply to fill in a file, a brief interview with prefabricated questions that expect prefabricated answers, with no opportunity to explain a bit about yourself because "we don't have very much time" …

When a psychiatrist visits a patient in a hospital ward, in the office of a rehab center or a private clinic, what does he have to deal with?

How important is empathy and how important is technique?

Another problem that afflicts psychiatric services in the public sector is the high turnover of qualified psychiatrists. There are many reasons for this: burnout, short term contracts, personal problems, but the fact remains that the patients are obliged to tell their story many times over in an attempt to establish a relationship with the new doctor, only too aware that sooner or later they will have to start over again. On their part the psychiatrists tend to concentrate more on diagnosis and treatment than on actually listening to the patient.

Another issue that cannot be ignored is the ever-increasing presence of social networks. Psychiatry should be based on listening and dialogue between two persons sitting one in front of the other. The social networks have eliminated the dimension of the body and have speeded up communications, eliminating distances. The psychiatrist can use Whatsapp to keep updated on the clinical conditions of the patient but must never forget that the ethics of the profession require their physical presence in meetings with the patients.

3. *Violence in psychiatric patients and in the man in the street*

This book recounts stories of people affected by mental illness who have committed crimes. Some were ill when they committed the crime, others were diagnosed with the illness after the crime was committed and the illness was considered to be the catalyst of their actions, others again became ill in prison and so were sent to the FPH. In all these cases the illness is linked to the crime, to an act of violence. A psychiatric assessment established the presence of a mental deficit, total or partial, but severe enough to render the person unfit to face trial.

Procedures apart, it is interesting to examine the link between psychopathology and violence. How serious must a delusional disorder or menacing auditive hallucinations be in order to affect cognitive processes to such an extent that violence results? Impulsivity plays a significant role in *Fiorenzo's* story; so when does impulsivity explode into violence? Does psychosis provoke more violence than neurosis, or vice versa?

And what about the violence committed daily by the man in the street? Murders, gang killings to settle scores, sexual abuse on minors, feminicide, not to mention suicide, the most extreme form of self-harm. Are all the perpetrators of these acts of violence mentally ill? Or are there mechanisms in the mind, such as aggressivity, that manifest in various levels of expression, from neurotic conflict—that only disturbs the balance of the person involved—to the act of violence committed against another person.

4. *Substance abuse and violence*

Eight cases out of the nine recounted in this book involve a comorbidity between substance abuse and mental illness.[30] In a systematic review, S. Fazel and colleagues[31] found that when substance abuse is associated with mental illness, the risk of violent acts increases. In the reflections on *Fiorenzo's* story, there is an evident connection between cocaine and the increase in impulsivity, while the comment on "*Lapo's*" story considers the function of self-medication by cocaine and alcohol, which however only aggravates the lack of emotive control and the anger, culminating in violence in the family context.

[30] Beneduce, R. (2013). Illusioni e violenza della diagnosi psichiatrica. *Aut aut*, 357, 187–211.

[31] Fazel, S., Gulati, G., Linsell, L., Geddes, J. R., & Grann, M. (2009). Schizophrenia and violence: systematic review and meta-analysis. *PLoS medicine*, *6*(8), e1000120. https://doi.org/10.1371/journal.pmed.1000120.

It is well known that drugs and alcohol contribute to cognitive distortion and disruption of the state of mind, and the cases commented on in this book confirm this. Psychiatry sees many patients affected by the so-called *double diagnosis* (a psychiatric disorder accompanied by substance abuse). They arrive in a phase of acute intoxication and evident psychopathological disorders such as induced psychosis; the drugs inevitably cause serious biological damage and a decline in their cognitive functions, and these patients, most of whom are very young, end up in rehabilitation centers with psychopathological profiles similar to those of schizophrenics. Like the FPHs in the past, the REMS receive and will continue to receive an increasing number of these double diagnosis patients; considering the damage that substances cause to the brain, one of the major problems these institutions have to face is how to rehabilitate criminals whose cognitive faculties (and not only) are so badly damaged?

5. *Diagnosis: a support for the therapy or simply a label?*

Giancarlo's story throws light on the role of diagnosis in psychiatry. In medicine it is an essential step towards identifying the correct therapy for the patient, but in psychiatry it plays a different role. As Roberto Beneduce said, it is "an epistemological weakness and a performative power". In other words, the diagnosis is a label that helps to define the patient's psychopathological condition. There are various ways of reaching a diagnosis: using the biomedical model with the DSM-5 manual, doing a classic diagnosis with phenomenological psychopathological categories, or taking a psychoanalytical approach for a structural diagnosis. Once the problem has been diagnosed, the objective is to support the patient throughout the therapy, including monitoring the prescription of antipsychotic drugs. Long term psychiatric patients are frequently diagnosed with different, sometimes very different, disorders during their illness, with the result that they end up taking multiple drugs (polypharmacy). Or it may happen that after suffering from an intellectual disability in childhood with comorbid psychiatric disorders, the patient is diagnosed with schizophrenia which marks them for the rest of their life; diagnoses that alternate over time, diagnostic errors, and psychopharmacological therapies prescribed to treat the symptoms, not the disorder. Probably the epistemological weakness of the psychiatric diagnosis derives from the complexity of the mind, which is not reducible to a biological datum. Furthermore, diagnosis also has a performative power, for example in cases where it is used in an assessment or certification. A diagnosis can radically change a person's life.

6. *Treatment for foreigners*

What happens to people affected by mental disorders who find themselves in difficulty in a foreign country? *Arthur's* story describes some of the difficulties that can be encountered and the progress that psychiatry has made in this area.

Ethno-psychiatry, the relatively new discipline created by combining psychiatry and anthropology, aims at providing culturally sensitive treatment for the mentally infirm of other countries. This requires a knowledge of that other culture, its traditions, religion, and rites; of how the disorder is perceived in that cultural panorama, which symptoms are seen as normal behavior and which are considered as being indicative of a disorder. As in psychiatry, listening to the patient is fundamental. Frequently there is a language barrier that makes a direct patient-psychiatrist relationship impossible, and the services of a cultural mediator are needed. This of course raises the question of the role of this professional figure. Is it sufficient for this person to translate what the patient says, or should they have some notions of psychopathology in the country of the patient so as to be able to empathize with their experiences and provide specific details if necessary?

For many years now, migration has been of great concern. In Italy, specialized structures have been set up, dedicated to the reception of immigrants arriving by boat or on foot. As Jacques Lacan remarked,[32] "Our future as common markets will be balanced by an increasingly

[32] Lacan, J. Originally appeared as "Proposition du 9 octobre 1967 sur le psychanalyste de l'Ecole", *Scilicet* 1(1968): 14–30. English translation: https://lacancircle.com.au/wp-content/uploads/2017/11/Proposition_of_9_October.pdf.

hard-line extension of the process of segregation" and indeed, these structures could well be considered as such extensions.

In addition to the trauma of arriving in a country where everything is foreign, language, climate, customs, food, migrants with only an alphanumerical code on a bracelet as identification, are obliged to recall the horrors of the country they left and the horrors of the journey they undertook, simply to obtain permission to stay. The ethno-psychiatric services of the Mental Health Department take on those migrants who are affected by a mental disorder and attempt to understand the treatment they need. The foreigner suffering from a mental disorder is by no means exempt from the risk of committing crimes and when this occurs, they are subject to the same treatment as the local patient.

3

The Forensic Psychiatric Hospital of Reggio Emilia

The Forensic Psychiatric Hospital of Reggio Emilia

Reggio Emilia, situated in the north of Italy, has played an important role in the history of psychiatry in Italy; the psychiatrists who worked in its two psychiatric institutions, the historical *Ospedale Psichiatrico San Lazzaro* (San Lazzaro Psychiatric Hospital) and the *Ospedale Psichiatrico Giudiziario* (Forensic Psychiatric Hospital) developed an interesting collaboration.

During the XVIII century, Francesco III, Duca d'Este, ordered a psychiatric hospital for the mentally infirm from Modena, Reggio Emilia and the surrounding countryside to be built on the site previously occupied by a leprosarium. It was commonly known as the *the general premises of the Mad House of the Estense States*. In 1821, Francesco IV, Duke of Modena and Reggio, well aware of hospital's limitations and shortcomings, nominated a young doctor from the city of Reggio Emilia, Antonio Galloni, to the post of director. It proved to be a far-sighted choice. Galloni took as a model the *Reali Case de' Matti*, the psychiatric hospital in Aversa, which at that time was under the enlightened direction of its

J. Santambrogio, *Stories from Italian Forensic Psychiatric Hospitals*,
https://doi.org/10.1007/978-3-031-61129-2_3

first director, Giovanni Maria Linguiti, introducing important changes such as abolishing the more brutal of the institutional practices, improving the hospital's living quarters and encouraging training courses for the staff (the *servants*). He also started to compile a psychiatric nosography and introduced Linguiti's so-called , i.e. treating the patients by accustoming them to discipline and work, but also allowing them to go for walks, participate in cultural activities and organizing summer breaks for them. Following Galloni's death in 1855, San Lazzaro fell into a period of decadence until the arrival of two prominent professors of psychiatry, Carlo Livi and Augusto Tamburini, both of whom improved the quality of the treatments and of the research being carried out at San Lazzaro. Inspired by the new trends and discoveries of positivistic science, and armed with the scientific equipment available at the time, they pursued research into the organic causes of mental illness. They also instituted systematic interventions to develop and perfect the hospital; in their view, similar to Galloni's, it was to be gradually transformed into a treatment center, in which the mentally ill would be exposed to discipline and education, instilling them with *a firm and direct will and conscience*.[1] This, in particular, was the line of action developed and proposed by Carlo Livi.[2]

Carlo Livi (1823–1877) was one of the leading figures in the field of psychiatry of his time. He was nominated to the chair of Forensic Medicine and Hygiene at the University of Siena in 1859 and in 1873 was called to direct the San Lazzaro Psychiatric Hospital. That same year he participated in the XI Congress of Italian Scientists in Rome and played an important role in drawing up the constitution of the Italian Society of Psychiatry. Two years later he founded the *Rivista sperimentale di freniatria* (Review of Experimental Psychiatry).

His successor, Augusto Tamburini (1848–1919), studied medicine at the University of Bologna; after graduating, he became First Assistant at the Civil Hospital of Ancona, after which he transferred to San Lazzaro,

[1] Paolella, F. (2020). La Gazzetta del Frenocomio: un esperimento di "giornalismo psichiatrico" al San Lazzaro di Reggio Emilia (1875–1881). *Rivista Sperimentale Di Freniatria*, *2*, 141–155. https://doi.org/10.3280/rsf2020-002008

[2] Tagliabue, L. (2013). Il valore di un Museo della Psichiatria a Reggio Emilia. *Rivista Sperimentale Di Freniatria*, *2*, 95–112. https://doi.org/10.3280/rsf2013-002008

where he studied under Carlo Livi. In 1876 he was nominated to the chair of Psychiatry at the University of Pavia and on the death of Carlo Livi in 1877 he became director of San Lazzaro, a role he then held for thirty years until 1907. His fields of interest included the border between mental illness and crime, non-imputability and treatment for the mentally ill who commit crimes. In 1876 he published a leaflet entitled "*Dei manicomi criminali e di una lacuna nell'odierna legislazione*" (Of Forensic psychiatric hospitals and a hiatus in current legislation) on the *Rivista di Discipline Carcerarie* (Prison Discipline Journal), in which he asserts that there are traits in delinquent madness that require particular forms of treatment and that such treatment cannot be comparable in any way with that meted out in normal prisons or even in civil psychiatric hospitals. The field of criminal madness was practically unexplored at that time, so grouping patients who had committed a crime together in the same institution offered the opportunity of studying the phenomenon and carrying out clinical observation. In Tamburini's view, in addition to criminals with mental illnesses, three main criminal categories should be interned in Forensic psychiatric hospitals: those who commit crimes for which it is difficult to establish a motive, whether they are driven by morbid impulses or perversity; patients with scores in the intermediate range of the Maudsley Personality Inventory (difficult to categorize between crime and madness) and patients suffering from recognized illnesses such as intellective, affective and impulsive monomania, and moral madness. He held that criminals suffering from mental illnesses or people suffering from mental illnesses who have committed crimes should be separated, the former in Forensic psychiatric hospitals, the latter in residences for the dangerously insane.[3] The fundamental concept common to these considerations, with its resulting institutional-organizational transformations, could be condensed into one word: dangerousness. "These patients, whether completely insane, or only partially insane, or abnormal and so unredeemable, were a source of perplexity and contradictions for a science that could only ascertain one thing about them: their dangerousness. The Forensic Psychiatric Hospital would protect them from prison,

[3]Tamburini, A. (1876). Dei Manicomi Criminali e di una lacuna dell'odierna legislazione. *Rivista di Discipline Carcerarie*, pp. 442–445, TO00194072.

which would have been a worse fate, while protecting society from their violence. It was a compromise."[4]

The law should have continued to provide for these people even if they had been judged as non-imputable, being of unsound mind (GBI–Guilty But Insane). In what way? By ordering that the person be hospitalized or interned in an appropriate structure until such time that the Forensic authorities issued new instructions. The prison system would physically contain the dangerousness and psychiatry would treat it.[5] Tamburini drew inspiration from the indications regarding the "Moral and Legal Status and Placement of the Criminal and Dangerously Alienated" issued by the International Medical Congress held in Brussels in 1875. The final *transactions* as they were called, stated clearly and unambiguously "M. de Smeth read the conclusions of the labors of the Eighth section, "On the Moral and Legal Status and Placement of the Criminal and Dangerously Alienated. (1) The section declared that in countries where the number of the condemned alienated is sufficient to create a complete hospital service, it is expedient to completely separate that class of patients. (2) By adopting the conclusion of M. Semal, the section expressed the wish that, in all other cases, those patients remain mingled promiscuously with the other alienated, and submit to the regime of surveillance and isolation necessitated by their mental state and the security of their surroundings."[6]

During Tamburini's tenure at San Lazzaro, a Forensic Psychiatric Hospital was instituted in 1892 to house the insane who had committed a crime, rather than having them sent to prison. It was the third institute of its kind in Italy after Aversa (1876) and Montelupo Fiorentino (1886). The imposing building in which it was housed had been constructed in 1675 as a monastery for the Fathers of the Congregation of the Mission

[4] Babini, V.P. (1981). Alcune osservazioni su una terapia ottocentesca: I Manicomi Criminali. Del Pistoia, L, Bellato, F. (eds), *Curare e ideologie del curare in psichiatria*, Maria Pacini Fazzi Editore, Lucca.

[5] Manfredi, M. Il Manicomio Giudiziario in Italia. Thesis in History of Psychiatry, relator Prof. V.P. Babini, Alma Mater Studiorum, University of Bologna, Academic Year 2012–2013.

[6] Resumé of the transactions of the International Medical Congress at Brussels, 1875. pp. 4–5. 101702097.nlm.nih.gov

(the Vincentians), suppressed by Napoleon Bonaparte in 1796 and converted into a prison.

Treatment for the insane and the dangerousness of the criminally insane and persons who commit crimes while of unsound mind was of great scientific and intellectual interest; Italy was active on the European front and was well represented at the international congresses.

By the end of the 1800s, Italy had 124 mental health facilities, of which 43 were publicly run asylums, but there was no legislation disciplining the sector. Given the number of mental health facilities and the scientific interest in the field, a law was finally passed in 1904, of which Augusto Tamburini was one of the prime movers. The law established certain fundamental principles: the director was given full authority over management and administration, and conditions for admissions and releases, conditions based on an inextricable bond between the Forensic authorities and psychiatry and between mental illness and the danger posed to society by the mentally ill. This law delegated responsibility for the treatment of most of the patients who had committed a crime to the Psychiatric Hospitals; these patients were confined to special sections or wards. One such was created in the San Lazzaro hospital and was known as *padiglione Lombroso* (the Lombroso pavilion). This law remained in force until 1930 when the *Codice Rocco* (the Rocco Code) modified certain measures and established that the mentally ill who had been acquitted of their crime, those who had gone mad in prison, were semi-infirm or waiting for trial should be interned in structures known as OPG (*Ospedali Psichiatrici Giudiziali*—Forensic Psychiatric Hospitals).

During the 1900s the management of San Lazzaro was deaf to stimuli from the fields of psychoanalysis, phenomenology and, in later years, sociology. Its organization remained rooted in the defense of the lunatic asylum structure, considered as useful *treatment*. Even the winds of change that swept in from Gorizia in the 1960s with the initiatives driven by Franco Basaglia and his colleagues were initially met with resistance. However, Giovanni Jervis, nominated Director of the *Centro di Igiene Mentale* (Mental Hygiene Centers) in 1969, did manage to start the process of innovation. In a first summing up of his new experiences, he stated, "The choices that led to the foundation of the Regional Psychiatric Service in 1969 were very clear. It was a question of providing an alternative to internment in lunatic asylums; to make a concrete contribution to extending the debate and the struggle against segregating institutions; to pave the way for bottom-up growth (in factories, neighborhoods, urban areas) for types of intervention and community management in the fields of psychiatry, medicine and health support".[7]

However, San Lazzaro was not closed down after the passing of the Italian Mental Health Act of 1978 (also known as Basaglia's Law after its principal proponent, Franco Basaglia), it even maintained a dominant role in the overall strategy of the psychiatric services of the Reggio Emilia region. Although it no longer took admissions, its survival on a symbolic level represented the reaffirmation of the need for a place in which to segregate and control difficult cases. Finally, with the arrival of a new General Director of the Health Services in 1997, the 230 inmates who still remained in the hospital were discharged and the building was reconverted to be used in the network of the territorial Services and Structures.[8] In this shuttling back and forth between the civil and the Forensic hospitals, in 1991 the inmates of the Forensic Psychiatric Hospital of Vicolo dei Servi were transferred to the prison complex in Via Settembrini, where a special section was set up for the mentally ill who had committed a crime, those who were awaiting trial, and the prisoners who had become mentally ill in prison. Twenty years later, in its report of October 2011, Associazione Antigone[9] described the Forensic Psychiatric Hospital in these terms:

"Similarly to the prison next door, the structural conditions of the Forensic Psychiatric Hospital have been negatively impacted by the scarce quality of the building materials used (leakages and dampness are evident in many areas). The cells are poky and frequently dirty, full of furniture and the personal possessions of the inmates. The inside bathrooms are old, narrow and badly in need of repair; they contain only a washbasin,

---

[7] Jervis, G. (1974). Cinque anni di attività dei Centri di Igiene Mentale della provincia. *La Provincia di Reggio Emilia*, 5.

[8] Tagliabue, L. (2013b). Il valore di un Museo della Psichiatria a Reggio Emilia. *Rivista Sperimentale Di Freniatria, 2*, 95–112. https://doi.org/10.3280/rsf2013-002008

[9] Associazione Antigone is a cultural and political NGO that operates to support rights and guarantees in the penal system. In 1998 it received a special authorization to visit prisons from the Ministry of Justice, after which it established an Observatory on Italian prisons. The Observatory now publishes an annual Report on the Italian penitentiary system.

toilet and foot basin and only cold water on tap. Due to overcrowding in the only section that is not used for healthcare, some of the cells house up to three inmates, two of whom sleep on a bunk bed, which is not an ideal solution given the nature of the inmates. The shower rooms are also in a very bad state and badly in need of repair: the tiles are filthy, and the floor and the walls are constantly damp due to a serious problem of condensation caused by the complete lack of aeration. Showers will be installed in the cells in some of the wings; work will start in December 2011. Since 2007 the structure has been operating as a *Casa di Cura e Custodia*,[10] a Rehab and Detention Center. In the past two years there has been a significant increase in the number of drug addicts held in these structures as probation sentences are very rare. The Forensic Psychiatric Hospital of Reggio Emilia has undertaken a praiseworthy experiment of leaving the cells open during the daytime; this program was first implemented in the Antares wing, followed in October 2009 by the Fenice wing. The experiment has been positive and the management is planning to extend it to the Andromeda wing, but not to Centauro, which houses inmates under psychiatric observation, coming from other penal institutes. The inmates from the wings involved in the experiment can leave their rooms but not the structure, and the prison guards are responsible only for the "security of the perimeter of the building". Only nurses and healthcare assistants operate in the sections involved in the experiment. The Centauro wing houses prisoners from other penal institutions, all the others sectioned patients. Another positive point worthy of mention is the hiring of medico-psychiatric staff. Now the structure has permanent psychiatrists hired by the local health authorities, whereas before it only had one internal psychiatrist and two externals for six hours weekly, so a constant

[10] The Italian penal system provides for internment in a "casa di cura e di custodia", a "rehab and detention center". These structures are a hybrid of treatment and detention. They are intended for the mentally ill who have committed a crime, for chronic alcoholics and for deaf-mutism. More precisely:

- persons suffering from mental illness and retained in custody for offences committed with criminal intent, for chronic alcoholics and for deaf-mutism;
- persons retained in custody for crimes perpetrated while under the influence of alcohol or drugs;
- persons retained in custody for other reasons, if suffering from a mental illness that does not require detention in a Forensic psychiatric hospital

presence could not be guaranteed. This has definitely improved the level of health care that the structure is able to provide, guaranteeing the constant presence of a psychiatrist on each wing and continuous checks and monitoring of the inmates' state of health. It has also had a positive impact on the admission process for new inmates, who now are given a psychiatric interview on arrival, whereas before this was done in the twenty-four hours following admission.

Medical staff: 1 healthcare director; 6 psychiatrists; 3 doctors; doctors on call (on twenty-four-hour shifts); 32 nurses (who provide a twenty-four-hour service); 20 healthcare workers (OSS); 5 rehab staff (hired during 2011).

The ratio of psychiatrists versus prisoners/sectioned patients is 1 for every 40 patients."

At the end of January 2014, when the law establishing the closure of the Forensic Psychiatric Hospitals had been passed and there was only one year to go before their transformation into the new Residences, I spent a week in Reggio Emilia meeting with medical staff and inmates, and creating a photographic reportage with the assistance of Caterina Clerici, a photojournalist. I kept a diary of this week, recording impressions and emotions; the entries for the week are summarized here.

Diary of the Visits

January 27: Day 1. Today is the start of a new, shared adventure into the realms of human relationships! The Director, Paolo Madonna, who has kindly agreed to see us, listens attentively while smoking one of his slim cigarettes. He introduces us to Chief Inspector Vito Bonfiglio, a Sicilian from Trapani with a kind face. He accompanies us on a tour of the various wings of the structure: Pegaso, Centauro (the wing that was not included in the open-door experiment), Andromeda, Fenice, Antares, and Cassiopea. We meet P., a sectioned patient in a cell at the end of the corridor. He has been keeping his door closed for some time now but doesn't really know why. Suddenly he starts talking in English with Caterina; he even dedicates a poem to her. Then we have an appointment with Dr. Valeria Calevro, the Chief Medical Officer since the Ministerial

Decree of April 1, 2008; before that she was the sole Director of the Forensic Psychiatric Hospital. We meet in her office to discuss the objectives of our project. After this meeting we continue our tour with Chief Inspector Bonfiglio, who explains the importance of the work done by the prison guards in the FPH; their role differs from that of the guards in a regular prison as it has a therapeutic aspect. He tells us about his relationship with Fiorenzo, who has spent twenty years in various prisons and FPHs. *Fiorenzo* has come to respect the guards, and after much work building relationships, he no longer sees them as enemies. Now we are in the Cassiopea wing, where there is a bar and a recreational area. Here I meet *Lucio*, who I had encountered previously in the psychiatric hospital in Monza. He is grateful to the guard who saved him when he attempted to commit suicide by cutting his throat in prison. He has an interesting history. At the end of the day we share our impressions with Dr. Madonna and then go to the Center run by don Daniele Simonazzi, the chaplain of the FPH and founder of *Il Grembo*, a structure that offers accommodation to the poor, to foreigners and former sectioned patients from the FPH, where we will stay for the duration of our visit.

January 28: Day 2. Inspector P. is waiting for us at the gates of the FPH. He tells us that a guard will accompany us to the *headcount*. This ritual takes place every morning at 8 o' clock. It is both visual and vocal: the guard has to make sure that all the sectioned patients are in their cells and, most important of all, that they are alive. Once an inmate was found hanging, his head in a noose, but there are also cases like that of Z., whose life was saved because the guard decided to do the headcount a quarter of an hour earlier that day. Z., a twenty-year-old from the Veneto region who hacked his father to death, is infinitely grateful to the guard.

After the headcount, we see another ritual, this time in the Centauro wing, where the high security sectioned patients beat the bars of their cells. No one has ever escaped from Centauro by filing the bars but it is well known that in other institutes the average time for doing this is twelve minutes.

January 29: Day 3. Interview with relatives. I meet N.'s mother and then take part in her meeting with her son. A very intense experience.

They touched the cords of a tormented mother-son relationship, creating moments of tension that I tried to defuse. N. was interned in the FPH following an complaint, probably out of proportion to the offence, that his mother "happened" to lodge.

Then I have another interview with *Fausto*, the poet. This is a moment of serenity and careful listening. We have lunch in the cafeteria and then have a meeting with a psychiatrist who tells us about the experiment in the Antares wing that started in 2000. This is an open wing with its own health staff, where the surveillance has been relaxed and they are working on constructing *psychic space groups*. The objective is to experience the transformation of the totalitarian institution to a place for treatment. An experiment that has become a laboratory. We go up to Antares where we meet *il Rasta* who is having a cup of tea. We interview a number of patients. Then we return to the Center, where we interview don Daniele. We receive a phone call from Monica Franzoni, actress and theatre director and coordinator for the FPH's theatre projects. She wants to meet us and skips dinner to come to talk to us. Then we go to the theatre to see a play put on by the patients. C. speaks of the pain of the responsibility for his crime. The mentally infirm are still responsible for what they do. He murdered his mother and sister.

January 30: Day 4. Breakfast at the Center then off to the FPH. The second coffee of the day and then up to Antares. We interview *Mario*. He shows us photos of his dogs and tells us his story. I can sense a deep distress, a distress that has taken form over time. Drug abuse (LSD) and hallucinations, the accident and the order to pay compensation. Why is he here? A simple case of obstructing an officer in his line of duty? There are some very emotional moments. Don Daniele arrives with a bag of gifts for us. A convivial moment with a young sectioned patient and a friend who has just become a father. I have a chat with P., who has spent more than twenty years in FPHs. He committed a murder. Caterina and I go different ways; she heads off with the guard to Cassiopea and then to Centauro. I have a meeting with Dr. Calevro. It's three o' clock. Our work here is finished. Dr. Madonna gracefully declines to be interviewed; he says that the patients have said everything there is to say.

Fausto: Madness and Creativity

Drug Abuse and (Il)legality

Now this is how I see it: if drugs are banned in Italy, why are they still easy to get? People get punished because they can get their hands on them. This is hugely immoral. If I can get it, it's likely that I'll use it. If I can't get it, I won't use it. That's my opinion, but I'm not a drug addict and never have been. Sure, I smoked a joint or two when I was fifteen or sixteen, but then I gave it up… now lots of other people, just because they can … like the proverb says, "Opportunity makes a thief".

When I was smoking that first joint, I said to myself, "Wouldn't it be better if I didn't?" Later on I went through much worse… It's only logical, if you can't get the stuff you don't say, "I want to get high, need to get high!". But here in Italy today all the kids smoke joints and yet it's against the law. Who knows if it's the State's fault for letting it circulate. Why do politicians and the State make these rules if they can't enforce them? Here in the FPH there are lots of people who take drugs, have taken drugs, who have been put in prison for years because of drugs. Let's put the responsibility for this on the two sides of the scales: I don't know who should be in prison and who not… the State who indirectly condones drugs, or the people who actually use them, or maybe both? Get it?

No, it's not my case at all. I gave up smoking joints. First, because I didn't get a kick out of it anymore, second because smoking a joint here means killing off someone 800 kilometers away. People kill for drugs. Here you only see a few grams being passed around, out there it's kilograms, tons and then it gets distributed on the open market. That's more or less what I think. If they made it legal, well, then it would be legal, right? The State should accept its responsibilities, that's the least it should do, no?

I have had a rather difficult life. I've always managed to come out on top of the difficult times because people care about me and have cared for me in the past. I'm here now because a doctor told me that I had to, that I could stop taking medication. I've been on treatment since 1994, I asked for it myself, because they poisoned me. They put LSD in my beer.

The beer, that was OK, it's food of a sort, it's good but I don't drink it anymore because I'm on medication; I was drugged against my will, I made a real bust up. I hallucinated, it was pure madness. I stole a car from a dealers: I drove it out, had an accident, ran away, got caught, got taken to police headquarters, then to hospital, then back to police headquarters, then to the reformatory in Treviso. I was seventeen and a half and I spent eighteen years there. I asked them to send me to the FPH because I had to be tied hand and foot. I was incredibly strong, I did sports, I got prizes in the Italian Greco-Roman wrestling championships. Yep. I was incredibly strong and just couldn't control myself. I had this flash of lucidity and asked the assistants to get me into hospital. They were really great and said, "Look, OK, we'll get you in". It took a heck of a long time … so I was in a pharmacologically induced coma. Sounds funny, but when I fell asleep I weighed 68 kg and when I woke up I weighed 106. I fell asleep with just some fuzz on my face, when I woke up I had a full beard. For starters they took me to Castiglione delle Stiviere, which in those days was nothing like what it is today. They made me sleep because that was what I wanted, but the treatments, the shocks, the hallucinations, I had them sometimes. That was in 1994–1995. I was being treated by a doctor that I wouldn't have trusted with a rag doll, let alone a human being. After ten years or so I was able to get away from him because I went to a Center because *something else happened. I got on fine* in this Center for three and a half years: I behaved myself, took the medication, had a great relationship with the psychiatrist… I'd say to him, "this medication, the dose is too high, this one here, the dose isn't high enough". He helped me a lot, he trusted me, he trusted the relationship we'd built up: "after all, what does it cost you? Here we are in a Center… if you tell me all about it, about how the medicine makes you feel, if it makes you feel better then I'll give you a bit more…" it wasn't really so *mercenary* as it sounds, well, maybe just a bit. We had a great relationship, he stopped giving me the jab because I felt much better, it got so I was just on maintenance therapy. Then got out, I went to Trentino, I'm from there and in Trentino there are lots of possibilities because it's an autonomous region and in my opinion they have too many resources… they should get some more competent people, more staff, "ah, that guy over there is his cousin…". There's a bit of mafia there too, because in Italy if you don't know the right people you're a nobody. You don't find employers with the same commitment that there once was, or workers with the same sense of pride in their work.

If you do your job fairly well, then that's ok, and that's why things are a bit approximate.

I arrived at Castiglione in 1994, they say it was in October and I stayed there until the following January, January 25. Then I went home to my mother. I don't have a father. We are three brothers, all with the same mother, but with three different fathers.

My mother was great. She looked after me, cared for me. My mother, she rocks, really rocks because she's got it together, you know… She's always stood up for me. And with me being in this situation and knowing all what my mother did for me, well, I get a lump in my throat, and sometimes I cry and I close up inside and I think "holy shit!".

When I was living at home I had to attend the Mental Health Center in my town for two years.

I woke up in the morning and went there every day. It took me from forty-five minutes to an hour and a half to climb two flights of stairs because although I've got the structure, I was carrying a lot of extra weight. I slept a lot and then there were the sedatives… it's not something that you can say, "it'll pass, it'll get better". Without the jab I lose weight and I almost feel better. But I let the doctors get on with it, it's their job after all.

I've spent seventeen years in and out of Centers and in and out of my mother's house. She and I have two completely different characters. In between Centers I worked, I like working, it satisfies me mentally.

I've done lots of jobs: mechanic, commercial traveler, carpenter, metal worker, caterer, pizza chef, cook, barman, dishwasher, gardener… I've done a bit of everything.

They sent me here from home. I'd finished a course of treatment, where they said, "yes, yes, he's fine, he's fine!". This psychiatrist, and he wasn't the lowest of the low, believe me, told me I could stop the therapy. Then I had a breakdown, and well, I did something … there was this other person.

Yes, well, ok, he was a pedo … but all the same… he was a human being that I have on my conscience. Eh, I killed him.

I Write Poetry Because I've Read the Dictionary

A typical day for me is I get up at 7.30, make some coffee, have breakfast. I shave every other day. I get dressed, I wash, take my medication and go down to the theater. I can't be doing with relationships here, these people are almost all drug addicts, lunatics, weirdos. I can't get on with people like that. No one teaches us how to get through life, we have to work it out by ourselves, these people just take advantage. Addicts, the whole lot of them.

I'm not judging anything or anyone. How could I, in my situation? I'm not asking for the moon. I'm here in Antares, I get on well with the doctors here. I've got a good relationship with don Daniele too. He's a good man, don Daniele, the *good don*! I'm off to his parish this afternoon to take part in a play with the FPH theater company.

About the treatment, well, I didn't really understand it at the beginning, but it's fine now. Leponex, Depakin, Haldol depot jabs. I quite like it here, it's an optimal setup. I work, study, do theater.

I write from time to time. I started when I was at home with my mother. She kept a room for me, all for myself. I painted and wrote. That was how I communicated with the doctor in the beginning. Ten years trying to communicate with a doctor that wasn't worth a brass farthing. A form of communication between me and me. What I'm turning into, what I am, what I'll be. Makes me think of the Alien in *Avanti un altro*.[11] I started writing poetry by chance. The first one I wrote was *Cinque passi* (*Five steps*).

Five steps
One more. Two steps.
One more. Three steps.
I contort with the earth's pain,

If I were slower
I'd see my eyes fill with color
I've destroyed too many dreams of innocence.
I've plundered innocence

[11] *Avanti un altro* was a popular television show aired on the Mediaset channel. The Alien was a popular character on the show whose opening comments were: [...] *who are you, where are you, where do you come from, where are you going.*

till only one veil is left.
Now, after five steps, I'm leaving the wonder and the trophies
to the God who created me
and did not embrace me.

Then there is this other poem I wrote about Castiglione delle Stiviere in 1994. I called it *Manicomio (Madhouse)*

Madhouse
A room
All white
No bench

A washbasin
All dirty
No water

A man
All silent
No sanity

Silence
All OK
No words

There were these people stuffed full of drugs in this hell hole. Because it was the old Lunatic Asylum in the town of Castiglione. The writing helped me, through writing I created memories of something that belonged to me and that was growing. I'm what I am because I wanted to be what I am. We are the sum of everything that happens to us, that's the truth of the matter. If something goes wrong, it leaves its mark on us; if it goes well, it makes us feel good. Don't know who said it, it's hearsay, but I say "I agree".

It's difficult to build relationships here. In one way or another, the whole world of psychiatry violates you. It violates you mentally. Because talking to the doctors means you have to explain your private thoughts to them. If you don't answer the questions you shut up, but if you shut up all the time, you clam up first and then you die, because humans are made to live in groups.

The psychiatrists usually listen to everything, however there are psychiatrists who understand and are able to give something more back; this is both dialogue and trust. Then there are psychiatrists that you talk to, but it goes in one ear and out the other.

Digging into the things that happened to you, isn't necessarily a bad thing, but you can't know a person's past. It seems absurd, but take a specific moment in time, X… in a minute after X I'll be completely different … and going back to that moment in time isn't easy.

Here's a good one, do you mind?

Benessere (Well-being)
I live the present, building the future
forgetting the past sometimes time wasted
balancing between the real world and the dream world
I live and that is riches in itself.
Standing up I realize how many times I fell down
and how many times I got back up
because falling is not failure
Failure is not getting back up.

I liked it, that's why I wrote it. I got the idea of writing poetry because when I was a kid I read the dictionary, twice I read it. Now I've forgotten it. All that knowledge, I'll have to put it somewhere.

Getting back up. Fall once, fall twice in a row, you're not likely to fall a third time. It's important not to give up. If you want to get back up, you will. It's the falls, the relapses, that leave scars on a patient's life. But the psychiatrist can help. If he's a good psychiatrist. If he doesn't care, or has off days … well…

We Are Fragile and We Create Masks

Mental illness is when you leave the straight and narrow. That's all it is. In my experience—I don't know if I was hallucinating or not—mental illness is when you come out with certain ideas … you leave your body behind. It's a bit hard to explain. When you do things that other people don't do, it's mental illness but only up to a certain point. Mental illness starts when you deviate. Take Einstein, for example: everybody studies mathematics but he created a real formula that was completely out of the box. Now, if he had done something just as out of the box, but in a negative way, then he would have been mentally ill too... do you get what I mean?

We live in a world where we are all fragile, we cover ourselves up to hide what we really are, we make lots of masks and shields. If a person doesn't know his condition, he's at a disadvantage because he has no way of knowing how he'll act in a given situation; after, like I said before, sometimes we are one thing and a moment later we something completely different while when we're faced with a situation we need to be tough, I think. We are human beings and we make mistakes. When the time comes for the reckoning, we have to reckon with ourselves and with other people. I can stay here, I can't stay here, what's the point of me being here? The question for all psychiatric patients, and not only for them, for everybody, is, "what do you want from life?". You can have lots of things from life, but if you don't know how to savor them and enjoy them in the right way, there's no point to them.

I'm not at ease with myself, because having someone's life on my conscience ... I'm doing my best to do good things, however I've got to pay off my debt as well as pay my way. It's tough having someone on your conscience, because you never know ... I had this moment of madness, what could I have done after? Hang myself? Die? When my time comes, I'll die too ... we all die. I've got something on my mind, do you mind if I tell you?

"We are alone when we are born, alone when we die, and in the middle? What a ballbreaker!".

Reflections on Fausto's Story

What is the nature of Fausto's interest in drugs, in the cannabinoids, for example? It has all the characteristics of a political battle against the State that doesn't legalize their consumption but still allows their use and assumes "huge responsibilities"—the fight against drug abuse and organized crime—but isn't able to shoulder them. Fausto's views originate in the context of the FPH, where the fact of living in close proximity with *other inmates* who have had, or are still having, problems with drug abuse, makes him particularly sensitive to and aware of the problem. In fact, he *only* tried a joint while the others are all drug addicts. It is interesting to see that he sides with the good guys, as opposed to the bad guys represented by the State and the other inmates, which could be one of the typical themes of the psychosis.

His whole psychiatric history appears to be linked to drug consumption. He says he was poisoned by LSD he involuntarily drank in a glass of beer and which would have induced a psychotic symptomatology resulting in behavioral relapses (the theft of the car); in addition, his presence in the FPH is connected to the interruption of the medicinal therapy he was taking which led to a further worsening of his symptoms, culminating in the murder. We have his version of the story: "[…] they poisoned me. They put LSD in my beer". How much of this statement is fact and how much is paranoiac? Could it be that Fausto took the LSD of his own accord, driven by a protective mechanism that would then attribute the responsibility for his behavior and the blame to the Other (the "Other of relationships" in the Lacanian sense of the term)? And could this same mechanism be involved in the case of the psychiatrist he accuses of having stopped his medication and so provoking the relapse? If this is the case, then it may be that Fausto himself intentionally stopped taking the medication, a common occurrence among psychotics. According to Fausto, his was the driving force behind his admission to the FPH because "I was incredibly strong and just couldn't control myself" and here the *body* dimension immediately comes into play, expressed as the physical force of a Greco-Roman wrestler. Here the psychosis is not only an aberration of the processes and contents of thought, but includes the relationship with the body. The Roman psychiatrist Bruno Callieri (1923–2012)—together with Danilo Cargnello, Francesco Basaglia, Lorenzo Calvi, Arnaldo Ballerini and Eugenio Borgna—introduced the concept of phenomenological psychopathology to Italy. He considered himself to be a doctor-philosopher, and on the question of the involvement of the body, remarked:

> The experience of one's own body (the lived body) is one of the essential cruxes of psychopathology and is one of the most enthralling problems of anthro-phenomenological research [...] we can say, with Sartre,[12] that my body is not a body, it is a tool-among-tools. It is irreducibly and originally mine because it is one with the being that I am. My body is imbued with subjectivity, it is a body-as-a-subject, not just a schema, "I am my body".[13] This clarification requires a mention of the distinction between *Leib* (the living body that experiences worldly things) and *Körper* (the material, anatomical body); the two terms express this fundamental difference classically.[14] We move constantly between the two poles of *having a body* and *being a body*, in existing, in being present, in Heidegger's fundamental concept of *Dasein*.[15]

During the physical and corporeal crisis that Fausto described, when, in the grip of a spurt of uncontrolled energy he goes to the car showroom, steals a car, has an accident, runs away, gets arrested, he is living his *Leib*; the *Körper* dimension comes into play when he asks to be "bound hand and foot". He transits from the active to the passive perception of his body, trusting in this latter perception that finally others will take over and look after him, and will ease him through the crisis.

Fausto himself describes mental illness as "distress that comes out of the body". Just as somatic illnesses have symptoms and indications at corporeal level—for example, running a temperature can be a sign of inflammation or the presence of a tumor—mental illness also has very clear bodily symptoms, such as a range of anxiety conditions, during which the patient experiences a sensation of constriction of the chest, tachycardia, that verges on panic and leads to a fear of death, or states of impulsiveness and aggression, when, like Fausto, the patient feels the presence of "an incredible strength that is impossible to control". In his

---

[12] Sartre, J.-P. (2003). *Being and nothingness* (H. E. Barnes, Trans.; 2nd ed.). Routledge.

[13] Marcel, G. (1967). *Metaphysical Journal.* Regnery Publishing. SBN-13: 978-0895269621.

[14] Galimberti, U. (1983). *Il Corpo*. Feltrinelli, Milan. p. 131.

[15] Callieri, B. (2007). *Corpo Esistenze Mondi*. Edizioni Universitarie Romane (our translation).

book, *Arcipelago delle Emozioni*, Eugenio Borgna[16] explores the relationship between mental illness and the body, focusing in particular on the changes that take place during puberty. "The mental picture of the body can warp into a *Stimmung*, a mood of rampant anxiety, to the extent of losing personal identity. The tendency (the impulse) to look in the mirror, desperately, time and time again, in the illusion of erasing, of seeing what is perceived as a defect dissolving, bears witness to this collapse (this debacle) of historical (personal) identity. We are in the area of disturbances relating to the consciousness of the *io* as Karl Jaspers used the term [...]. Things become even more complex and ambiguous: not only do I live this body in a state of dissociation and disintegration, it is no longer *my* body: as the borders that separate it from the social-world and the environment-world are lost, it becomes the [possible] body of others. Indeed, here the body is no longer the receptacle of subjectivity and intentionality; it is sucked down into the vortex of the dissolving of the consciousness of the io and that of the body, both eroded by dissociation and disintegration. In certain cases, the split of the consciousness of the body, that finds its expression in the radicalization of the dilemmatic existential structure of adolescence, cannot be stemmed, nor can it be compensated, except by the onset of ravings which would appear to originate in the context of this split between the io and the body."[17]

In addition to commenting on the experience of the changing body in adolescence, in this same volume Eugenio Borgna also speaks of other psychopathological experiences regarding the body, such as vital feelings of sadness, psychotic depression and schizophrenia, in which latter case the perception of the body changes. "Patients do not experience the body as decomposing, or disintegrating; indeed, it maintains its unity and compactness but its significance fades. It dwindles into the distance, it is no longer knowable or graspable, it is unknown. The body is present in consciousness as a fact of consciousness but it is no longer an immediate

---

[16] Eugenio Borgna is a professor at the Nervous and Mental Illness Clinic of the University of Milan, a position he has held since 1962. From 1970 to 1978, he was Director of the Psychiatric Hospital of Novara; since 1978 he has headed the Psychiatry Service of the Ospedale Maggiore of Novara. He has studied, in particular, the psychopathology of depression and schizophrenia.

[17] Borgna, E. (2001). *L'arcipelago delle emozioni*. Feltrinelli, Milan, pp. 99-100 (our translation).

experience. For example, it is possible to perceive (recognize) the sound of one's own voice, while not accepting it as belonging to one's body."[18]

Eugenio Borgna recalls the writings of Klaus Conrad[19] to describe the experience of feelings of strangeness and ethereality of the body that in extreme cases can be perceived as decomposition and disintegration, with a loss of borders vis-à-vis other people, culminating in the silence and immobility typical of catatonic schizophrenia. In his book, *Come se si finisse il mondo*, he comments:

"This state can lead to the loss of continuity and historicity of the body: certain body parts can still be perceived, but others not; hence the terrifying experience of existing as a split-being and a lacerated-being: a being slumped in the abyss of the body's decomposition and disintegration. The origins of disorders of articulation of movement and gestural expressions present in the catatonic *Lebensweld* would appear to be linked to changes in the experience of the body, that after all are also interwoven with changes in the experience of the io."[20]

Another important theme that Fausto develops in his reflections is the doctor-patient relationship, or to be more precise, the *psychiatrist-patient* relationship. He wouldn't have trusted the first psychiatrist, in whose care he remained for approximately ten years, "with a rag doll", while the relationship with the second psychiatrist, who worked with him at the Center, is excellent. "He helped me a lot, he trusted me, he trusted the relationship we'd built up" to the point that they modified the dosage of Fausto's medication on the basis of how he felt. Finally, he mentions a doctor, a chief psychiatrist, who he asserts told him he could stop taking his medication that resulted in him "having a breakdown, and well, I did something" to another person. Fausto's opinion regarding psychiatric therapies are interesting, "In one way or another, the whole world of psychiatry violates you. It violates you mentally. Because talking to the doctors means you have to explain your private thoughts to them. If you don't answer the questions you shut up, but if you shut up all the time,

---

[18] Borgna, E. (2001). *L'arcipelago delle emozioni*. Feltrinelli, Milan, p.105 (our translation).

[19] Conrad, K. (1958). *Die beginnende Schizophrenie. Die beginnende Schizophrenie. Versuch einer Gestaltanalyse des Wahns*. Thieme, Stuttgart.

[20] Borgna, E. (1995). *Come se finisse il mondo*. Feltrinelli, Milan, p. 81 (our translation).

you clam up first and then you die, because humans are made to live in groups. The psychiatrists usually listen to everything, however there are psychiatrists who understand and are able to give something more back; this is both dialogue and trust. Then there are psychiatrists that you talk to, but it goes in one ear and out the other. Digging into the things that happened to you, isn't necessarily a bad thing, but you can't know a person's past. It seems absurd, but take a specific moment in time, X… it'll be different in a minute … and going back to that moment in time isn't easy."

Fausto's view of what could be a good psychiatrist-patient relationship is echoed by Eugenio Borgna in his book, *Arcipelago delle emozioni*: "The only way to practice psychopathology and psychiatry is to get the patients to speak and bring their anxieties and suffering back to the surface […] The only way to come closer to [the patient's] interior life and the interior regions of their suffering is to listen to them, to try to construct a dialogue that is not aridly clinical and permits the two participants to engage in a context of reciprocal opening-up and liberty of expression (shards of liberty are to be found even in psychotic experiences)."[21]

Fausto's ideas of what constitues "a good psychiatrist" are very similar to those expressed by Glen Gabbard, cited in Chap. 1 (page xx).[22] To develop the therapeutic rapport with a psychoanalytical approach, Gabbard describes how it is possible by observing the dynamics of the transference and countertransference to plumb the depths of the doctor-patient relationship: during transference the patient tends to reconstruct his internal world and psychiatrists do the same.[23]

Fausto gives the impression that in his experience with the psychiatrist (indeed, the psychiatrists) there is an undertone of violence, violence suffered, in the sense that his vicissitudes, his stories, his innermost and most intimate thoughts and doings, were "laid bare". True, the psychiatrist was in a position of possessing both knowledge and know-how, so there was a state of asymmetry between the two. The psychiatrist, the *good*

[21] Borgna, E. (2001). *L'arcipelago delle emozioni*. Feltrinelli, Milan. p. 103 (our translation).

[22] Gabbard, G.O., Roberts, L. W., Crisp-Han, H., Ball, V., Hobday, G., Rachal F. (2012). *Professionalism in Psychiatry*. American Psychiatric Publishing, Washington D.C. p. 12.

[23] Gabbard G. O. (1995). Countertransference: the emerging common ground. *The International journal of psycho-analysis, 76 (Pt 3)*, 475–485.

psychiatrist, who knows how to listen and is "able to understand and give something more back", is able to see and live the contradiction of their "superiority" and knows how to divest themselves of it at the appropriate moment and suspend judgement, in order to enter into a state of harmony with the patient's true self, and own.

According to the Italian psychopathologist Gilberto Di Petta, "only the *epochè*, the suspension of judgement, is the key to the breakthrough, the magic touch, the act of un-anchoring that only in a state of authentic empathy allows access to the apparent obviousness of the unthinkable, where Lorenzo Calvi,[24] with delightful simplicity, tells us that "it is still possible to be in the condition of discovering something"".[25]

Gabbard, writing this time on the necessity of training, provides a valuable insight; he notes that psychiatrists are in a privileged position with respect to the patient, the relationship is in fact not symmetric. It is essential that the psychiatrist is careful not to exploit this position of power in the therapeutic relationship; indeed, the training for psychiatrists leads to exhaustive auto-examination.[26]

What Fausto describes regarding his experiences with his psychiatrists inevitably leads to a question regarding his encounter with us. We sat at a table, and Fausto began to talk freely about himself and read his poems. Maybe he felt he had found fertile ground? a good listener? The standard questions: "Would you like to tell us about yourself?", "What's your opinion of the FPH?", "What is life like, here in the FPH?", "What is mental illness?", were intended to provide a support to encourage any answer, intuition, or desire to tell. Given Fausto's response, I believe there was indeed a *meeting*. Something happened that went beyond the guidelines of the standard questions. Fausto wanted to talk about himself, and we listened. We approached Fausto with the desire to meet, and what he told us, he told us because we wanted to know. This meeting certainly threw light on routine psychiatric practice! The ability to listen has been lost, psychiatry boils down to collecting data instead of stories and

---

[24] Calvi, L. (2005). *Il tempo dell'altro significato*, Mimesis, Milan (our translation).

[25] Di Petta, G. (2008). *L'ultima lezione in Io e Tu, fenomenologia dell'incontro*. Edizioni Universitarie Romane, Rome. p. 147 (our translation).

[26] Gabbard, G.O., Roberts, L. W., Crisp-Han, H., Ball, V., Hobday, G., Rachal F. (2012). *Professionalism in Psychiatry*. American Psychiatric Publishing, Washington D.C. p. 18.

communications, there is no longer the will to hear what the patient is really saying, instead words are put into their mouths, to correspond to what is required from them.

Fausto distinguishes between good psychiatrists and bad, and the difference lies in the quality of the listening and the ability to "give something back", and that "something" is dialogue and trust.

And indeed, Fausto's creative vein originates in this need to communicate: "I write from time to time. I started when I was at home with my mother. She kept a room for me, all for myself. I painted and wrote. This was how I communicated with the doctor in the beginning. Ten years trying to communicate with a doctor that wasn't worth a brass farthing. A form of communication between me and me. What I'm turning into, what I am, what I'll be". When he isn't able to express himself in speech, he communicates through words that provide images of his situation. Writing is an instrument that helps him know himself and helps other people to know him. His collection of poems reveals a beauty and delicacy of language, with images of nature, such as ripples on the river, sun, flowers, rain, grey skies (*I contort with the earth's pain*), of places (*Hospital, Madhouse*), relationships (*Mirroring me in my eyes*, *The age of friendship*, *Chasing the stranger*), of hope (*Well-being*), of love (*Destiny, I love you*), his relationship with God (*Five steps*) and this poem:

> *My love*
> Poetry
> is instinct
> you can caress it with thought
> you can feel it between the heart and soul
> or just touch it, simply, with your hands.

Fausto uses free verse to communicate his poetry.

In *Hospital* and *Madhouse* he describes the reality of the places in which he has lived. A spiral of hope connected to the visit of his doctor, the hope of a change, emerges in the verses of *Hospital*:

When I am in this room / hope lives / I leave the door ajar / to hear footsteps / doesn't matter, almost nothing / of the hell or infinite /

paradise with a smile, / I hear a footstep / of the judgement of the doctor / there is no time my heart thumps / vegetable soup and mashed potatoes / all the rest takes care of itself.

Madhouse ends with the eloquent image of "silence no words": silence by nature is without words, but in reality silence could "speak", could communicate something. If the silence in Fausto's *Madhouse* has no words, it is an indication that this place has annihilated humanity and suffocated subjectivity.

Well-being is an ode to the courage of hope. Here Fausto is aware of his "relapses in psychiatry", understands the errors in his past and with a dose of sane realism says we can only live in the present ("I live and that is riches in itself"), with a glance directed to the future and "because falling is not failure / Failure is not getting back up".

The conclusion of *Five steps* that talks of his relationship with God is of significant interest. "Now, after five steps / I'm leaving the wonder and the trophies / to the God who created me / and did not embrace me." Why would God, after creating him, reject him? He communicates the image of a fruit that is born, grows, matures and then is harvested. But God creates and then rejects. Here Fausto seems to be hinting that God's relationship with man is virginal, estrangement. A God that leaves space for freedom. God does not harvest, does not use, does not exploit mankind, he simply creates humans and gives them liberty of action and thought. The words of Charles Péguy, in *The Mystery of the Holy Innocents*[27] comes to mind regarding the mystery of the freedom of mankind:

> Such is the mystery of man's freedom
> Such is the price we set on man's freedom
> Because I myself am free, says God, and I have created man
> in my own image and likeness.
> Such is the mystery, such the secret, such the price
> Of all freedom.
> This freedom of this creature is the most beautiful reflection in this world

[27] Adapted from the English translation by Ann and Julian Green. From *Basic Verities*, Books for Libraries Press, reprinted 1972. © by owner. Provided at no charge for educational purposes.

Of the Creator's freedom. This is why we give it,
and place on it, its true value.
A salvation that was not free, that was not, that did not come
from a free man could in no wise be attractive to us. What would it amount to?
What would it mean?
What interest would such a salvation have to offer?

Fausto speaks of a gift again in Destiny, in which the image of a flower is intertwined with that of the loved one: The flower is not forgotten / to be plucked or uprooted / Without sin, with great joy / it will come back / to show its color / or to be gifted to the first great love.

In his book, *Di armonia risuona e di follia*, Eugenio Borgna poses the question of whether illness of the soul gives rise to creative imagination. "Poetry comes into being, in spite of the presence of the illness: poetry is influenced in the positive or negative sense. But there can be alternations, or intermittences, in the ways in which poetry, or artistic creativity, encounter illness."[28] Writing about the correspondence between Nelly Sachs and Paul Celan, he states, "It is not the illness itself that gives rise to poetic creativity but the pain that is associated with it: as is well known, this is the ineffable thought of Leopardi and Simone Weil."[29] Finally, in another comment on the poetry of Nelly Sachs, but which I find applicable also to Fausto's, "Nelly Sachs' poetry would not have been what it is if it had not been nourished with fragility and kindness, sensibility and yearning, anguish and pain, that the psychosis—this epiphany of pain which is madness—amplified in its horizons of feeling."[30] These concepts are present in Fausto's poetry also: it was pain, nourished by fragility and sensibility, and not his illness, that inspired his poetic vein. The very style and logic of thought in these poems bear evidence that they were written during a phase of relative psychic stability.

[28] Borgna, E. (2016). *Di armonia risuona e di follia*, Feltrinelli, Milan. p. 43. (our translation).
[29] Borgna, E. (2016). *Di armonia risuona e di follia*, Feltrinelli, Milan. p. 48. (our translation).
[30] Borgna, E. (2016). *Di armonia risuona e di follia*, Feltrinelli, Milan. p. 53. (our translation).

Postscript

Nine years later, in November 2023, I was able to visit Fausto again and find out how he was faring. He was pleased to receive the visit and was happy to share his thoughts, which are reported below.

I'm fine now, thanks to the medication I'm taking. When I was in the FPH they found the right medication and I'm still taking it. This is very important. Knowing what a person needs or doesn't need, it isn't easy. The medication is important for me to be able to make progress. When I left the FPH I went to the REMS in Pergine Valsugana. I did voluntary work there, in a nursing home: I folded napkins, helped in the laundry. Then I started to work for a big social cooperative, on the production line. I was a bit freer, I had good support, I could go for a walk in the park with no problems. Then they sent me to this community because I worked hard and I was really willing to work and I could handle it… So, I spent three years in the REMS in Pergine, two and a half years in another community and I've been here for two and a half years now.

I really want to go and live by myself. But … there's a problem. When I killed that person, I was living alone. It was in 2011. I was living alone and I messed up, maybe I could have avoided it but, well I was smoking joints, drinking myself under the table every day. Everyone told me I was a mess. Evenings I would go from my village to another village, five kilometers on foot, I'd leave at half past eleven and get back home at five in the morning with the bus. That was my life in those days, I'd go walking at night, sleep most of the morning, get up for lunch, go to work. But I was living on my own. One day I don't know what got into me, I committed that crime. A really bad crime. But if I'm here, that means there's still a chance for me.

I would like… No, that's not right, would like is the wrong word, never use it, it's better to say I wish. Yes, that's it. I wish I could have a space of my own to share, a little apartment. Where I am now, I don't know if I can achieve anything. Four mornings a week I go to this social co-op, where they work wood. Look, this is a candle holder I made out of plywood. The parts are fitted together, dovetailed.

What can I say about myself? I like coffee and I smoke a packet of cigarettes a day. The other people here don't talk much. I asked permission to go out for a walk, because I think while I'm walking or I walk while I'm thinking. Unfortunately I can't go out alone, I have to wait for the report that says I can. I go to mass, I'm religious. My faith helps me, not the church so much, but my faith helps me stay in touch with the world. I feel my heart beating. I take communion every Sunday, but I don't confess. I talk to God, He's not in the church, He's behind everything, I see Him in the plants, on the mountain tops. The confession is between myself and me, between myself and God, the priests aren't interested in my sins, I don't need a priest.

I'm much better off here than in the FPH. They are two different places. The FPH is closed in. Something nasty happened to me there. One of the other inmates punched me and I fell down, then he kicked me when I was still down. I've forgiven him. You get to understand a lot of things in the FPH and in prison. There's a lot of social dangerousness around. It depends how you look at it and there's a lot to say on the subject, at the moment I don't feel I'm dangerous. I never felt dangerous. But it's not for me to say, there are many things in my life, a life full of bad mistakes. But I write poems. I wrote my first poem in the first year of middle school, then in 2000 I started to write properly. Poetry brings out the most important things, the search for an image. When I was in primary school, I got a dictionary as a prize and I read it through and through, I liked the words, and I kept on reading the meanings. I've always been an artist, a bit mad (but in the good sense of the word) and a bit self-destructive. I painted and worked clay. I modelled my hand in clay, it looked real. I don't know if you'll believe me but when I was four years old, I solved Kubric's cube. In 1987 I'd already thought up the electric car, with an engine that charges with an exchange of electricity. The idea came to me when I was fixing bicycles. I could do various things in my mind, with my intellect. It's essential to be able to communicate clearly. It's not what you say so much as how you say it.

I'll read you this poem that I wrote, I called it Psychiatry 2020.

I'm feeling low
Talk to me…
I'm talking

I'm feeling low
Listen to me…
I'm listening

I'm feeling low
Try to understand me…
Maybe I can feel your pain

I'm with you.

Davide: Paranoia and Crime

The Forensic Psychiatric Hospital Isn't Hell and I Don't Have Toothache

My experience with Forensic Psychiatric Hospitals started in May 1994 and continued till January 2006 when I was admitted to a rehabilitation center. I did a fair amount of damage there in seven years, so here I am, back in the FPH. But it isn't hell.

No, in spite of what you might think, it isn't hell. If you're objective about it and look at it from an intelligent point of view that I don't claim to, it's a branch of the system that does its best not to trash the desperate cases. In other times, folk like me, like us, would have been thrown out, isolated, they would have shut us up and thrown away the key, bye-bye. Here they try not to trash us.

Sure, the FPH, I've got a dirty word on the tip of my tongue, yes, the FPH could be the world's arsehole, hoping that they won't…

I'm exaggerating. This isn't hell, it's a place where folk like me, folk with problems, have a bed with blankets, heating, and food that you can eat. That's what I think.

If you're going to talk to the others, a lot of them will tell you the food's grim, that it's cold, it's hot.

I think you have to take care of the primary needs, and once you've got them, it's up to you to be happy. If you are pathologically unhappy, nothing will make you happy, not a FPH, not even a great rehabilitation center like the one I was in.

I've never been unhappy. And I don't have toothache either.

I remember that once during an interview, a psychologist asked me, "what's your definition of happiness?". I said, "having no pain". She was shocked, scandalized, "that can't be right!". It's right enough. Try having really bad toothache, when you get it sorted you'll see I'm right! But maybe you're interviewing the wrong person here because I don't have toothache and I'm happy. You're probably interviewing the least representative inmate of the FPH.

I Existed on Whisky and Cannabis

Before the FPH? As a child I was left to myself mostly. I was first in the class, right through middle school, due more to cunning than to work and study.

I got my diploma from the scientific high school, again more by cunning than by studying. And while I was at high school I started drinking, drinking far too much and as an adult I started taking drugs as well, experimenting here and there, getting a lot of bad habits too. And I wasn't happy. I was costing 500,000 lire a day and that didn't make me happy either. Then I was in care and taking psychopharmacological drugs… so my life before the FPH is just a haze, my young days are all fogged over and I thank God—because I am lucky enough to be a believer—that, in spite of having tried to bombard my health in every possible way, I'm feeling quite all right and can say that I'm happy here in the FPH. It's more God's success than mine.

It was drug abuse that got me involved with psychiatry. And then I didn't want to do military service because I had things set up at home, so I lived on whisky and cannabis in the barracks they sent me to. You can imagine what I said to the doctor there; well, to be honest I can't imagine it myself … then they sent me home and that's when my psychiatric pathway started. It went on till '87 when I tried to kill myself with an overdose of pills. I woke up in Diagnosis and Treatment[31] and that's when I started the psychiatric pathway I'm following now. I've been really lucky with the treatment I've been taking since October 1998. The doctor that started me on it was a real benefactor. I've been taking that treatment ever since.

My Home in the FPH

Two pills of Olanzapine a day, one at eight in the morning and one at eight in the evening, I don't know what it does but I do know what it doesn't do, compared with other much less pleasant psychopharmacological drugs. When I take it, I can play music, I can study, the quality of my life is much better than that of lots of people on the other side of these bars. I heard this story on the news about this couple, more or less my age, who went to shelter in a rundown building; the floor gave way under them and they fell into a tank of rainwater. They were found there two weeks later.

I'm a prisoner, imprisoned by bars and duties, obligations to respect the wardens, the nurses, healthcare assistants, the doctors, I'm a prisoner behind bars, the bars are my prison but how many people who are not behind bars are still prisoners, imprisoned by poverty or suffering? '*Io, vagabond che son io, vagabondo che non son altro*'[32] (Me, wanderer that I am, I'm nothing but a wanderer), well f**k that wandering nonsense, I'm much better off in the FPH.

It's cold outside for the 'wanderers that I am'. Maybe they have their faith, those 'Me, wanderer that I am, I'm nothing but a wanderer', but they'll be cold now. Sorry … excuse my anti-apocalyptic song digression.

At this moment in time the FPH is my home, a place where I feel welcome.

---

[31] Diagnosi e Cura: The 'Servizio Psichiatrico di Diagnosi e Cura (SPDC)' is a division of the Department of Mental Health, dedicated to the treatment of and assistance for people with critical psychiatric problems. It offers voluntary hospitalization, hospitalization for sectioned patients (TSO) and urgent consultation services.

[32] From the song by the Nomadi, '*Io, vagabondo*'.

A home. I was born, brought up, and lived in the family home, always in the same house.

It was 1993, I'm not going to bore you with all the details but that was when I got into trouble the first time… and from there, prison. I ended up in the hospital under observation and then in the FPH. That was 1993, twenty years and seven months ago. And after twenty years and seven months of drifting, 'home' for me is where I can lay my head down on a pillow, where I sleep, the people I eat with are my 'family'. This idea of mine of 'home' is rather improvised. I was in a rehab center for seven years, and that was 'home'. I try to treat my home well, I don't bite the hand that feeds me, I don't piss in the bed I sleep in.

A Therapeutic Relationship with the Warders

I hardly know anything about prison; I was only in the prison in Modena for three days and I was put in the hospital ward there after two hours as I had a history of psychiatric problems. I spoke to a doctor, and then to a psychiatrist and two days later I was in the hospital's prison wing. So I really don't know anything about prison at all.

I do know that they intimidate you as soon as you arrive, you get thrown into a cell with a blanket and you just have to hope that the tap works and there'll be running water. I was there for two hours, the atmosphere here is friendlier than the real prison atmosphere, here you can build a relationship with the wardens.

You've seen the place, haven't you? There is nothing traumatic anywhere here, I treat the people well who treat me well, and they treat the people well who treat them well, keeping the right distance and using respect.

I use the formal '*lei*' form when I speak with the warders, they can use the informal '*tu*' form when they speak to me. Those are the rules and I'm fine with that. In any case, the relationship with the warders… these are people doing their job and trying to do it well. If they do their best for everyone, their best is good for me too.

The quality of my life is improving, so… no, the warders have never done anything bad to me.

The relationship with a warder can be sort of therapeutic. But this happens everywhere, on the outside too, not just in the FPH. All relationships can be therapeutic; all relationships can be traumatic. What's traumatic can be therapeutic too, if it doesn't kill me, it'll do me good. What's therapeutic can be traumatic in that a pleasant therapy can turn into an unpleasant therapy, but when that happens you've brought it on yourself in one way or another.

I'm a Paranoid Schizophrenic

I've got my own idea about mental illness, it's my personal idea, very, very personal.

For me, mental illness isn't an illness like the 'flu when a virus attacks you, and then when the 'flu goes, the virus goes too.

You don't have a mental disorder; it's something that roots itself in your soul to the extent that you are that disorder. It's not that I *have* paranoid schizophrenia, I *am* a paranoid schizophrenic and I don't think that's a play on words.

It's something that's linked to your being. It's something that you are, not something that you catch, an illness caused by germs and things. Maybe, in a life as messed up as mine, or as unfortunate as that of many others, it's possible to be forced into becoming what we are, the mentally sick. Yes, you can be forced, or drawn, into it. However, for me the starting point isn't "I'll get rid of your schizophrenia for you". If we're talking about a starting point, for me schizophrenia is *confusion*, that's what I identify it with. While paranoid, well, I've been structurally paranoid since I was a boy.

I've got a problem with trust. I've got to keep people in my sights, I've a hard time trusting people. I think men are wicked, but maybe that's because I'm wicked myself. But about "being paranoid", I'm *paranoid*, it's not as if someone comes along and gives me a pill, and then I'm not paranoid anymore. It's structural, a question of mental architecture.

In the eleven years and eight months I've spent in the FPH, I've ransacked the library. When I was in the rehab, I ransacked Mondadori. This helped me be a little less schizophrenic, but I'm still paranoid.

Crimes Committed Out of Desperation

Paranoids, now I'm trying to speak for myself here, commit crimes out of desperation when they can't see another way out of the situation. The problem is that being paranoid, they see situations as being desperate even when they really aren't. In this case, objective and subjective are terms that play an important role. On the other hand, no one in this world can say how much of your thought is objective and how much is subjective. We are all tied to our own perception of reality and we do what we can, we don't perceive what we want, how and when we want. As believers, we perceive what we are given to perceive.

It's as if the mental illness, the disorder, alters the capacity, the lucidity, to see things as they really are.

I committed my crimes because I was convinced that that was the only way out. I was sure of it. That's it; the paranoid is sure, he isn't convinced, he's sure. Now that I know this, often when I'm in an acute state of paranoia and I become stroppy, I try to break out of my vicious circles—if I'm cold, I ask someone if it's cold or I try to see if I'm running a temperature that would make me feel cold rather than running around screaming "it's cold! It's cold" as maybe it's just my paranoia or a few lines of temperature that makes me say I feel cold.

Subjective and objective are two cogs in a gear that never fit together for anyone.

If I'm having one of my better days, I find it easier to talk to other people and find out if it's cold because a window is open or because I'm running a temperature. On bad days, when the illness has the upper hand, I can't do that and so I live in a world on my own.

And mental illness can be brought on, oh yes. Paranoia can be exacerbated by an unfortunate series of signals from the world, things that come from the outside, things you feel, an unfortunate series of events that make even a psychiatrist convinced that you're paranoid, even though you're not.

And yes, I read a bit of Axel, and I did drugs; don't mind me if I'm a bit *Matrix*, a bit *Truman Show*…

Hey, I've already forgotten the explanation I gave you of paranoia! If I only knew what paranoia really is, I'd be my old self again in five minutes.

I've given you some definitions that to me are honest, but it's only my point of view. I'm a paranoid and there are millions of paranoids, men who kill women, things like that, stalkers, that's paranoia.

I Popped as Many Pills as I Could

In the years before 1998, it would have been between 1994 and 1997, I changed therapies a number of times. I was a smoker, I popped as many pills as I could, now by the way I've given up smoking. Yes, I ate pills like they were sweets. Like any druggie who knows his stuff, happiness was having chemicals in my blood stream, so between 1993 and 1997 I took as many pills as I could get my hands on, thinking that I could sort myself out that way, with pills or drops, at that time the nurses let me have them, I smoked like the proverbial chimney, drank decaffeinated coffee; I felt a lot of compulsion and the therapies made me feel uncomfortable. I was distressed, I was, and the therapy didn't help, in fact, maybe it made things worse because a paranoid who is weakened by Haldol, a paranoid who feels like a herbivore weakened by Haldol surrounded by carnivores becomes even more dangerous because he feels weak. When you feel strong, the paranoia recedes, you've got more space around you, you can breathe better. When you feel weak, the fact of being paranoid and feeling weak, even a kid could kill me, well, let's say you feel worse.

I've tried other therapies too, not just anti-psychotics. To start with, relationships are therapeutic. I'm thinking of a psychologist and a psychiatrist in particular. The psychiatrist that took me on a year ago when I came back here, I cried when I saw him, but not because I'd been sent back to the FPH, but because I thought I'd end up with one of those doctors who hate lunatics, who throttle you with therapies and throw you into a cell and then throw away the key; but no, I got Doctor P., my benefactor, who prescribed Zyprexa in 1998 and before that Leponex in 1997, which made the situation better but not completely. But Zyprexa, that's a whole different ball game. If they told me, "You have to take Zyprexa for the rest of your life", no problem. I take my pills in the morning, I put them on my bedside table at night and I take them without anyone having to check on me because they don't bother me at all. If this is the price to pay for being paranoid, two 10 milligram pills of Zyprexa a day, I'm fine with it!

Danger to Society, the Fear You Cause in Others

This is no joke. What does 'danger to society' mean to me? I remember, it was 2004–2005, a meeting with a psychiatrist, two psychologists and all of us here in Antares. The psychiatrist, talking about danger to society said to me, "You know, Davide, with those unblinking eyes of yours, like two headlamps blazing away and that stare, not to mention your size, and evident strength, people could be afraid of you". For twenty years I'd been thinking of how afraid I was of other people, but I'd never thought they might be afraid of me. Danger to society, that's a fear of what you could do to others, what you could do to society. They keep us locked up because we are socially dangerous. Because society is afraid of us or maybe, as good paranoids, we are afraid of society. It's all about fear, about what you can do to protect yourself, keeping yourself safe, but that's impossible, you can never be safe, no one is ever completely in control, no one is safe. No one knows if they'll twist an ankle going through that door.

The future… on television too you hear songs about the future, but what do we know about it? And yet… I believe that from the artistic standpoint it's all marketing; there's a group of people who think that that is how it will have to be and they buy the disk. But apart from that … who knows what the future holds? And that business of danger to society? Now I'm going to blab on a bit about danger to society because I'm really not clear about it. I don't know if I'm a danger to society or not.

I think, if I'm treated right, I can treat others right too, as well as being good mannered. I think I love my fellow men as far as I'm able. With all my limits, of course. But then there are those situations where you start to close up, and then to isolate and when you're isolated you interpret reality as best you can because you are on your own without anyone to talk to, to compare notes with, so to speak, and that's when you become a danger to others, a danger to society. At least, this is what happens when you are paranoid; I'm speaking for myself, I don't know how it is for other diagnoses, I don't have the info.

American Coffee to Start the Day, a Good Moment

My typical day in winter goes like this: I get up around seven in the morning. I wake up, out of habit, I get up, get dressed, make my bed, I do all the things you do in the morning, and I try to be tidy because that helps too.

As schizophrenia is confusion, I try to keep things tidy and live in an orderly environment (I'm in a cell on my own) … I'm in Centauro. I see it this way, trying to live in a well-organized environment helps to keep the mind tidy too. I wash my face, try to make myself as presentable as possible and then I wait for the morning events to start, the therapy, breakfast, a cup of American coffee. When your last meal of the day is at seven in the evening, at seven in the morning anything more than water to put in your stomach is more than welcome. And anyway, that American coffee in the morning is always good. From November I can stay in this room or, if it's busy, I can go somewhere else; the guards are really good about that. I can play my guitar here on the ground floor for a couple of hours. And I really enjoy that. I just have to be careful not to meet other inmates… that's OK, everything's fine.

It just means that if someone comes in, I have to make them leave. Those are the rules and we have to take them as they are. I'm fine being alone so I don't have to play songs for all and sundry. And this is another way of keeping things tidy, studying music and so on. Music is a real passion of mine. I've been passionate about music since I was a boy and it helps me with my symptoms.

You could say that paranoia is an exasperation of opinion; music isn't an opinion, it's a system. It's a system on the theoretical level and technique on a practical level.

To play a piece correctly you need physical technique. Bach's cultural system is a constructed system, it's structured. Yes, there's no getting away from it. You don't play music with opinions. Pardon my platonic idealism. Going back to the order I was talking about earlier, music brings order, it helps. I think reading helps too, it could help me put things in order, I'm not going to cite authors and non authors, I'm not going to believe anyone else's truth, not even that of the Bible even though I'm a believer, but you can find particles of truth anywhere, even in the dumbest detective stories.

I've just started playing music again in the Church with Don Daniele but because I'm a believer and not an idolator I've got a problem with the temple. Let's say I'm a heretic, OK, they don't burn us at the stake anymore. We can talk about it. Even if I'm a heretic, they don't burn us at the stake anymore or at least, not for this.

The Theater and Moments of Glory

The relationship with Monica, I'll start from the beginning. Now, I think it was in the spring of 2004. I was in Antares, that's the open wing and I had a guitar. I was doing the cleaning, I was really busy and I heard about this theater laboratory Monica was running, at that time she taught stretching. The first meetings were clandestine, and we got away with it because the head keeper turned a blind eye. They were held right after lunch in one of the school rooms as there was plenty of room there and I remember that at that first meeting Monica said, "When acting, the first thing that those of us who come from Emilia Romagna have to do is to close our vowels, close those 'e's and 'o's at the end of the words." A question of pronunciation. OK. I thought this over a bit and I thought, "This brunette has her head screwed on the right way. She's got things to say". I went on going to the clandestine theater laboratory, but I kept my mouth shut, and when they started talking about some sort of show I said, "Me? Act? I can play the guitar!". And we managed to get something going with six guest actors—some read their parts, others knew them by heart—directed by Monica; the moron with the guitar sat in the corner at the back on the right and we managed to put on a piece entitled '*Who are the bad Guys*?'. It was made up of pieces taken from the in-house paper that at that time was called "Effatà', recited by the actors and accompanied by my guitar, original pieces, composed, but not really composed, just tiny snatches that lasted less than a minute to give a dramatic undertone to the action on the stage. Nietzsche was furious with Wagner because he said that everyone was capable of writing dramatic music. I wish I could compose dramatic music! I'd be more than happy with just that. I'd make Nietzsche mad. I had my moments of glory too. I think it was in October 2005. At the Cristallo, it was. I went to do our bit with the amplifiers and all. The audience was on its feet, the stage was two and a half meters deep, with a cinema screen right there. There we were, all in a line, and I remember that we brought the house down. That was a real moment of glory. We did it again on Palm Sunday 2006. They had set up a marquee in the big courtyard, and over 2500 people came. There was the RAI[33] too, and the audience applauded for three whole minutes, but it wasn't such a thrill as it had been in the cinema. What happened at the Cristallo was a real moment of glory.

Theater and music help me, you know. They are therapeutic.

Remember that song, the one by Fabri Fibra, "The more you dream, the less you do, the more you do, the less you dream"? So, if you do things as they have to be done or should be done, or if you try to improve them, you dream less and have fewer opinions. I know it's not very democratic but… I'm more for an intelligent dictatorship than for democracy.

The Future Is a hypothesis

It's not me that makes the future, it's the future that makes me. There's an exchange between me and the future. The future is a hypothesis. My Dad is ninety-three, tomorrow is his ninety-third birthday, he's at home and doesn't go out, but he's fine, he's all there up top, he's got a full-time nurse and he's fine.

The only relationship I have with the world is with my Dad and a cousin.

[33] RAI, Radiotelevisione Italiana—the national broadcasting company, owned by the Ministry of the Economy and Finance.

They treat me nicely, the situation is what it is, we do each other OK. They don't condemn me too much but they don't put me on a pedestal either. It's a good relationship.

My future? I haven't got a clue. I know that this afternoon, unless there's an earthquake of 12 on the Richter scale, I'll come back to my room and play the guitar in peace; if it goes well, I'll be content, and if it doesn't, I'll be frustrated.

Then I'll have a long afternoon. My bathroom light went out, so it'll be a bit dark, I can't read unless I go into the bathroom where there's neon lighting, so I'll watch television, what else can I do? MTV music and off we go! And boredom, I've discovered that boredom is a symptom.

It's a symptom of dissatisfaction. If you are left on your own and you begin to feel dissatisfied, boredom sets in. It's a form of self-torture. Boredom sets in which is a bad way of thinking in itself, but doesn't mean you are thinking bad things about yourself. I remember my last moment of boredom, the last two hours of boredom, in 2000 I think it was, but not because I've had lots of distractions, but because I've identified it, I think.

Reflections on Davide's Story

Everyone criticized the FPH, describing it as unacceptable, inhuman, to be closed whatever the cost, but here we have an inmate who says he is happy in this *hospital.* Davide's view of the FPH is interesting. He says he feels welcomed, taken care of, "it's a place where folk like me, folk with problems, have a bed with blankets, heating, and food that you can eat". He's aware of the fact he's imprisoned by bars and obligations, but not by poverty and misery. He defines it as "a branch of the system that does its best not to trash the desperate cases", a "home". How can we account for Davide's positive judgement?

Could it be that this is a person who has fallen on times so bad that even a FPH seems welcoming? However, this isn't a question of making a moral judgement on Davide's behavior. What interests us is discovering why certain inmates were happy there and could therefore be against the closure.

Davide encountered psychiatry due to substance abuse, having been sent to a psychiatrist following medical check-ups during military service. He admitted having used various substances including cannabis and spirits.

Particularly worthy of note is his attitude to religion in relation to his life, "I thank God—because I am lucky enough to be a believer—that, in spite of having tried to bombard my health in every possible way, at this point in time I'm feeling quite all right and can say that I'm happy here in the FPH. It's more God's success than mine." In addition to this he says he's taking an Olanzapine-based anti-psychotic treatment that improves his quality of life.

When asked about his views on mental illness, he made a perspicacious distinction between being insane and having a mental illness, "It's not that I *have* paranoid schizophrenia, I *am* a paranoid schizophrenic and I don't think that's a play on words." Unknown to Davide, this was the view taken by Ludwig Binswanger[34] and Jakob Wyrsch[35] who held that there is no such thing as schizophrenia, only the schizophrenic. Current, more politically correct usage holds that the person has a particular illness (he has schizophrenia) rather than being identified with it (he is schizophrenic), while Davide is not in agreement with this, reflecting on a question of identity and identification with the illness, "Paranoid is something I am structurally, I've been that way ever since I was a boy. I am paranoid, and it's not that someone can come along and give me a pill, and I'm not going to be paranoid anymore. It's a question of structure, of mental architecture." "You don't have a mental disorder; it's something that roots itself in your *soul* to the extent that you are that disorder."

Jacques Lacan, in Book 3 of his seminars, *The Psychoses*,[36] talking of the phenomena that make up *mental architecture*—the term Davide himself used—in a psychotic patient, stated that they are "as elementary as a leaf

[34] Binswanger, L. (1956). *Drei Formen Missglückten Daseins: Verstiegenheit, Verschrobenheit, Manieriertheit (Three forms of failed existence and its relevance for contemporary psychiatry)*. Max Niemeyer Verlag.

[35] Wyrsch, J. (1949). *Die Person des Schizophrenen: Studien zur Klinik, Psychologie, Daseinsweise*. Verlag Paul Haupt.

[36] Lacan, J., & Miller, J.-A. (Ed.). (1993). *The seminar of Jacques Lacan, Book 3: The psychoses 1955–1956*. page 19 (R. Grigg, Trans.). W. W. Norton & Company.

is in relation to the plant, in which a certain detail can be seen of the way in which the veins overlap and insert into one another—there is something common to the whole plant that is reproduced in certain of the forms that make it up. Similarly, analogous structures can be found at the level of the composition, motivation, and thematization of a delusion and at the level of the elementary phenomenon. In other words, it's always the same *structuring* force, as it were, at work in a delusion, whether it's the whole or one of its parts that is under consideration".

Davide's thoughts on mental illness, based as they are on his experiences, have a certain wisdom and depth, and are culturally intelligent: mental illness cannot be superimposed on a physical illness that we *have*, such as *having* a heart attack, *having* diabetes. Mental illness affects a person's entire being, their soul. It's something mysterious that spreads through a person's life, history, it envelopes their relationships, the things and people to which and to whom they are attached, their passions. To a certain extent, mental illness is unique.

The interview with Davide has opened a chapter on differential diagnosis between paranoid schizophrenia and paranoic psychosis or paranoia; indeed, it seems probable that he is suffering from the latter.

In his doctoral thesis (1932), Jacques Lacan posed the following questions: "Does [paranoid psychosis] represent the development of the personality, communicating a constitutional anomaly or a reactive deformation? Or should it be considered as an autonomous illness that, interrupting the development of the personality, recasts it?"[37] In his *Lehrbuch der Psychiatrie*, Emil Kraepelin wrote that he remembered when approximately 70% to 80% of the patients admitted to hospital were recorded as suffering from paranoia.[38] In those days, paranoia was the psychiatric term with the widest and least precise meaning,[39] in addition to which it was the least suitable for clinical use. In the 6th edition of his *Lehrbuch*, published in 1899, he first made the distinction between

[37] Lacan, J. (1932). *De la psychose paranoïaque dans ses rapports avec la personnalité.* Éditions du Seuil. Our translation.

[38] Kraepelin, E. (1883). *Compendium der Psychiatrie: zum Gebrauche für Studirende und Aerzt.* Metzger & Wittig.

[39] Séglas, J. (2012). *Paranoia: Systematized Delusions and Mental Degenerations. An Historical and Critical Review.* Nabu Press.

psychosis and dementia, describing paranoia as "the furtive development, resulting from inner causes, of a lasting, immovable delusional system that is accompanied by the complete retention of clearness and order in thinking, willing and acting."[40]

Jacques Lacan, however, criticized this definition in his third Seminar: "Its development isn't gradual, there are always surges and phases. It seems to me, but I'm not absolutely sure of this, that it was I who introduced the notion of fertile moment. This fertile moment is always visible at the beginning of paranoia. There is always a break in what Kraepelin goes on to call the progressive evolution of a delusion dependent on internal causes. [...] When one looks for the triggering causes of a paranoia, one always observes with the required question mark, an emotional element in the subject's life, a life crisis that in fact does involve his external relationships, and it would be astonishing if one were not led to do this with respect to a delusion that is essentially characterized as a delusion of reference—the term isn't Kretschmer's but Wernicke's."[41]

Davide defined himself as "paranoid schizophrenic" but he did not show any hallucinatory symptoms, disorganized speech, disorganized behavior or negative symptoms. His thoughts did show some bizarre traits, but without structured delirium, which can probably be attributed to the Olanzapine he was taking. We were not able to see his medical records or receive more detailed information about his history, so I based my diagnosis—with all its limitations—on the clinical presentation to the interview and the material that emerged from Davide's discourse. I found his phrase, "Paranoid is something that I am structurally", to be fundamental, indicating that he was more paranoid than schizophrenic.

In his book, *Trattato di Psichiatria Forense* (Treatise on Forensic Psychiatry), Ugo Fornari gives a synthetic clinical distinction—according to DSM-5[42]—between delusional disorder, paranoid schizophrenia, and paranoid personality disorder:

[40] Kraepelin, E. (1899). *Psychiatrie, Ein Lehrbuch fur Studierende und Artze.* Johann Ambrosius Barth.

[41] Lacan, J., & Miller, J.-A. (Ed.). (1993). *The seminar of Jacques Lacan, Book 3: The psychoses 1955–1956.* p. 17 (R. Grigg, Trans.). W. W. Norton & Company.

[42] American Psychiatric Association. (2013). *DSM-5, Diagnostic and Statistical Manual of Mental Disorders, Fifth Edition*, American Psychiatric Publishing.

(a) "The delusional disorder (297.1, DSM-5) is characterized by the presence of non-bizarre, interpretative or intuitive delusions, stable over a period of time, without hallucinations. As far as its exact nosographic collocation is concerned, this delirious disorder or syndrome includes paranoia, paranoid psychosis, and the sensitive delusion of reference".[43]

Therefore, the DSM-5 has included in the delusional disorder category, the *old* syndromes that phenomenological psychopathology characterized by the understandability of the delirium: paranoia and sensitive delusion of reference.

Tanzi and Lugaro, in their *Trattato delle malattie mentali* (Treatise on Mental Illnesses) written in 1905, defined paranoia as "…a constitutional anomaly that remains latent during youth and manifests in later years, taking the form of a slowly evolving, coherent and fanatic delusion that approaches the farthest limits of probability without crossing them, that feeds on every circumstance of life and is supported by a good memory, a unilateral but acute critique, a solid stubbornness to the clearest denials. Hence the delusion completely possesses the paranoid, identifies with his personality, and becomes the inspiration for his behaviour. The constancy of the paranoic convictions is brilliantly confirmed, if not by common sense, at least by determination and oft times the stoical dignity of life".[44]

In their monography *La vergogna e il delirio* (The Shame and the Delusion), Arnaldo Ballerini and Mario Rossi Monti explored the views of Ernst Kretschmer, professor at the School of Psychiatry of Tübingen, known as the founder of a psychiatric typology based on the study of the human constitution:

"In 1918 he described as a development of personality the onset of a delusional syndrome separate from schizophrenia, essentially because in schizophrenia the delusions are always bizarre and incomprehensible, and its evolution assumed to worsen. The sensitive delusion of reference has the characteristics of the psychological intelligibility of certain cases of paranoic psychosis. These are often

[43] Fornari, U. (2018). *Trattato di Psichiatria Forense*, UTET, Turin. p. 687. (our translation).

[44] Tanzi, E., Lugaro, E. (1923). *Trattato delle Malattie Mentali*, Vol. II, Società Editrice Libraria. p. 756. (our translation).

non-bizarre and well-organized delusions without hallucinations, that partially correspond to Kraepelin's paranoia.[45]

In fact, Kretschmer followed his paradigmatic cases for years, pushing the Jaspersian biological method of understanding by identification to the extreme, more as a possibility of following an evolution in an effort to "understand genetically" (Jaspers, 1913) rather than the possibility of reliving an isolated experience or a constellation of *Erlebnisse*. This form of "genetic understanding" delineates a common theme of significance that runs through a person's entire history, the world in which he finds himself and the world he builds, his models of characteriological functioning, his defenses and their failures. In this way a circularity of definition can be traced between the sensitive delusion of reference and intelligibility: a sensitive delusion is understandable, and it is defined as sensitive precisely because it is understandable. [...]. On the basis of subjective phenomenology, traditional psychopathology claims that a delusion is understandable (hence the definition of delirious) if the themes are in harmony with the directives of the emotive background.[46]

(b) In paranoid schizophrenia (295.90, DSM-5), on the other hand, auditory hallucinations and bizarre delusions (influence, transmission, theft or insertion of thought) are more evident and are not present in delusional disorders. In addition, affectivity disorders, disorders of the will and language and catatonic symptoms are not pre-eminent in paranoid schizophrenia.

(c) Delusions and hallucinations (Group A, personality disorders, DSM-5) are not present in paranoid personality disorders (301.0, DSM-5) as the disorder is fundamentally focused on suspiciousness, diffidence, the search for hidden meanings in other people's conversations and gestures, psychorigidity, extreme vulnerability, rancor and sensitivity. The paranoid personality differs from the schizophrenic in that it is not delirious."[47]

---

[45] Ballarini, A., Rossi Monti, M. (2011). *La vergogna e il delirio—un modello delle sindromi paranoidee*, Giovanni Fioriti Editore. p. 10. (our translation).

[46] Ballarini, A., Rossi Monti, M. (2011). *La vergogna e il delirio—un modello delle sindromi paranoidee*, Giovanni Fioriti Editore. P. 18. (our translation).

[47] Fornari, U. (2018). *Trattato di Psichiatria Forense*, UTET, Turin. pp. 687-688. (our translation).

Over and above the clinical characterization of paranoia, for which I have relied on the help of several influential authors and their seminal works, Davide's story leads us to reflect on criminal etiology, in his particular case on the relation between the structure of paranoic thought and the passage to the act or crime.

"Paranoids, now I'm trying to speak for myself here, commit crimes out of desperation when they can't see another way out of the situation. The problem is that being paranoid, they see situations as being desperate even when they really aren't. [...] I committed my crimes because I was convinced that that was the only way out. I was sure of it. That's it; the paranoid is sure, he isn't convinced, he's sure."

Once again, in the words of Ugo Fornari, "In the paranoic disorder, the passage to the act is promoted by the overlapping of a stenic stimulus and one of astenia (in the psychastenic) or by extreme susceptibility (in those with expansive personalities), which can be provoked by even slight external stimuli (an adversity, a reprimand, a slight, a misinterpreted gesture, etc.) but which clearly is subjectively abnormally processed. The dynamic or evolution of the reaction usually follows this sequence:

- A real event that is interpreted as an offence;
- Inability to react appropriately and satisfactorily;
- Passage to act.

In the delusional disorder, the primary criminogenic role is played out by delusional cues or by a delusion of objectification of various content and orientations, in the sense that the person suffering from grandiose delusions makes others suffer; the vigorous side of the person's personality greatly outweighs the depressive side, whereas the person suffering from the sensitive delusion is dominated by depression. The passage to the act in the context of illness represents the dissociative evolution or the brusque, improvised revelation of a delusion, so that the *persecuted* becomes the *persecutor*. This behavioural imbalance is often induced by depression when the delusion, in the evolutional phase, is not shared or approved by other people. In this case the passage to act may be directed against the person themselves."[48]

[48] Fornari, U. (2018). *Trattato di Psichiatria Forense*, UTET, Turin. pp. 690-691. Our translation.

When telling his story, Davide did not mention his crime specifically, but he did explain the dynamics that led him to commit it, and the conviction that there was no other option open to him, just as Fornari laid out in his sequence of the reaction dynamics.

At this point, the following comments on violence in psychosis by Martha L. Crowner are very much to the point.

"Many factors may explain violence in people with psychosis besides psychosis and other psychopathology:environmental factors, cultural, interpersonal and attitudinal factors; and other, unknown factors. Aggression is a universal human drive, the expression of which is shaped by social norms and external contingencies. In some circumstances the expression of aggression in assault can be adaptive. […] In a large survey of about 10,000 adults in the United States, the Epidemiologic Catchment Area survey (Swanson et al., 1990), subjects were classed as violent if they admitted to one of five behaviors within the previous 12 months: physical abuse of a child, physical fighting, physical fighting while intoxicated, fighting with a spouse or partner, and fighting with a weapon. […] The rate for those with schizophrenia was 13%, whereas for those with major depression it was 12%, for adults who abused canabis, 19% and for those who abused alcohol, 25%. […] In logistic regression analysis, male gender, youth, poverty, substance abuse, and major mental illness all predicted violence, as did the interaction between substance abuse and major mental illness. […] In a study of a diagnostically mixed population (Monahan et al., 2001) and in surveys of large community samples, Link et al., (1998) identified a relationship between paranoia, delusions of control and thought insertion (known as threat/control override), and past history of violence in both psychiatrically ill and control subjects. Arsenault et al. (2000) concluded that violence in subjects with schizophrenia was partly explained by excessive perceptions of threat. […] A study of 1410 patients in treatment for schizophrenia, a substudy of the National Institute of Mental Health Clinical Antipsychotic Trials of Intervention Effectiveness (the CATIE project; Swanson et al., 2006) explored the associations of violence and symptoms. Serious violence was associated with hostility (odds ratio [OR] 1.65), suspiciousness and delusions (OR 1.46), hallucinations (OR 1.43), grandiosity (OR 1.31) and excitement (OR 2.9). Delusional thinking alone was not associated with serious violence, but when it occurred with suspiciousness and persecutory delusions it was highly associated (OR 2.9). [...] In a forensic setting, Taylor (1985) found that the crimes of a group of men motivated by delusions were more serious than crimes of other psychotic men. He suggested that psychotic symptoms may frustrate men so they lose self-control and tolerance of others; in this way she proposed an indirect mechanism—that is, irritability or reactivity—through which psychotic symptoms can lead to assault.[49]

In addition, Davide adds another interesting concept regarding his pathology, *the relationship between objective and subjective*. This relationship involves the patient's internal and external world, as well as that of the psychiatrist who is looking after them.

"On the other hand, no one in this world can say how much of your thought is objective and how much is subjective. [...]. As believers, we perceive what we are given to perceive. It's as if the mental illness, the disorder, alters the capacity, the lucidity, to see things as they really are. [...] I try to break out of my vicious circles—if I'm cold, I ask someone if it's cold or I try to see if I'm running a temperature that would make me feel cold rather than running around screaming "it's cold! It's cold" as maybe it's just my paranoia or a few lines of temperature that makes me say I feel cold.

Subjective and objective are two cogs in a gear that never fit together for anyone.

If I'm having one of my better days, I find it easier to talk to other people and find out if it's cold because a window is open or because I'm running a temperature. On bad days, when the illness has the upper hand, I can't do that and so I live in a world on my own."

As Davide explains so clearly, in the world of the paranoic, the subjective dimension is amplified. His perception of cold might not correspond to the real temperature when measured with a thermometer. This is where the Other (in the sense of the Other of a relationship, in Lacanian terms) appears as a touchstone. When the paranoic accepts the existence of the

[49] Crowner, M. L. (2008). Schizophrenia and delusional disorder. In R. I. Simon & K. Tardiff (Eds.), *Textbook of violence assessment and management* (pp. 105–121). American Psychiatric Publishing, Inc.

Other, and is receptive to making a comparison, their mental state is positive but when they reject the Other, when the Other is perceived as a persecutor, the subjective experience becomes amplified and distorted, the *cold* becomes excessive and there is no possibility of correcting the perception with a comparison. For further reading on the subject of the relation between *percipiens* (the person who perceives) and *perceptum* (the object that is perceived) in psychosis, the reader is referred to Jacques Lacan's *On a Question Preliminary to any Possible Treatment of Psychosis.*[50]

The psychiatrist, too, constantly experiences the critical aspects of this objective-subjective relationship in his work. What will be the objectivity of a patient who has been the victim of violence? And how much of what this patient recounts can be considered subjective? To what extent can the psychometric tests quantify the objectivity of the patient's experiences? How does the subject-doctor organize the cure for the subject-patient?

Giuseppe Sabucco and Sergio Carlì wrote about the peculiarities of psychiatry compared with other medical sciences and the complexity of the patients in their article *L'odore della diagnosi* (The smell of the diagnosis) published on the Melegnano hospital house organ, *Quaderni di psichiatria pratica.*

"It is paradoxical even to call *object* that which constitutes his/her interest as psychic suffering definitely has a subjective side, and it is evident that expressing "a psychological concept in the first or third person implies evidence criteria that are not homogeneous, as in the third person (*he* is depressed), the psychic state is identified by observation of behavior, while I don't need to observe my behavior to establish that *I* am depressed. In this case it is a grammatical passage that highlights different ways of experiencing" (U. Galimberti, 1996).[51] So, no brain imaging can completely illustrate the specific "different ways of experiencing" for that patient, our object but his subject, and the visit to the psychiatrist is, inevitably, a meeting of two subjects. Throughout the twentieth century this characteristic of the psychiatric sitting has been investigated both by

---

[50] Lacan, J., Sheridan, A., Bowie, M. (2001). On a Question Preliminary to any Possible Treatment of Psychosis. Routledge. https://www.taylorfrancis.com/chapters/edit/10.4324/9781003059486-6/question-preliminary-possible-treatment-psychosis-jacques-lacan-alan-sheridan-malcolm-bowie.

[51] Galimberti, U. (October 5, 1996). Vi accuso cari psicologi. In *La Repubblica.*

phenomenological thought and by psychoanalysis. Both found that the intersubjective meeting is unrepeatable".[52]

Given his psychopathological condition and the crimes committed, Davide was acquitted and assessed as being socially dangerous. His own correlation between his paranoia and his state of social dangerousness is interesting as it encompasses the possibility of a double prospective, internal and external, subjective and objective.

He recalls a significant episode when a doctor told him that "he could frighten people".

"For twenty years I'd been thinking of how afraid I was of other people, but I'd never thought they might be afraid of me. Danger to society, that's a fear of what you could do to others, what you could do to society. [...] They keep us locked up because we are socially dangerous. Because society is afraid of us or maybe, as good paranoids, we are afraid of society. It's all about fear, about what you can do to protect yourself, keeping yourself safe, but that's impossible, you can never be safe, no one is ever completely in control, no one is safe. [...].

I don't know if I'm a danger to society or not. I think, if I'm treated right, I can treat others right too, as well as being good mannered. I think I love my fellow men as far as I'm able. With all my limits, of course. But then there are those situations where you start to close up, and then to isolate and when you're isolated you interpret reality as best you can because you are on your own without anyone to talk to, to compare notes with, so to speak, and that's when you become a danger to others, a danger to society. At least, this is what happens when you are paranoid; I'm speaking for myself, I don't know how it is for other diagnoses, I don't have the info."

Davide talked at length on the theme of individual fear also in the context of his paranoia; for further reading on this topic, the Italian philosopher Danilo Zolo wrote an interesting text, *Sulla paura. Fragilità,aggressività, potere* (On Fear. Fragility, aggressivity, power)[53] in which he explores fear and aggressivity in individual and collective contexts, comparing various authors such as Arnold Gehlen who was the first

---

[52] Sabucco, G., Carli, S. (October 1999). L'odore della diagnosi. In *Quaderni di Psichiatria pratica*. Melegnano Hospital internal house organ, UOP 33, (p. 30). Our translation.

[53] Zolo, D. (2011). Sulla paura. Fragilità,aggressività, potere. Feltrinelli.

to write explicitly on the relationship between fear and aggressivity[54] and Konrad Lorenz, one of the founders of the science of ethology (Nobel prize, 1973) who also wrote on the subject of intraspecific aggression.[55] According to Gehlen, men are oppressed by a perception of fear that not only can make them aggressive, but can turn them into murderers, while this does not occur, or at least, only marginally, in the animal world.

On the question of the fear Davide mentions as indicated by the State and perceived by society, that same fear he had never thought about but which the doctor pointed out to him, two Italian criminologists, A. Ceretti and R. Cornelli, suggest interpretations on the "grounds of the current security policies with the objective of giving them a democratic orientation, in the ambit of a project for a civil and open society that is able to transcend fear in coexistence".[56]

When attempting to define what social dangerousness means to him, Davide starts from his own subjective experience (frightening other people, being frightened), omitting the other side, the objective definition given by the experts and the court, as not being within his area of competence.

Article 203 of the Italian Penal Code states that a person is socially dangerous when they have "committed any of the indicated facts, even if they cannot be charged or punished for them… and it is probable that they will commit new facts that the law establishes as being crimes. The traits of the socially dangerous person are inferred from the circumstances indicated in art. 133." Obviously in the case of a psychiatric assessment, the expert pronounces on the social dangerousness related to the mental disorder (psychiatric social dangerousness), and not on other types of social dangerousness.

Once social dangerousness has been ascertained, security measures are applied. These measures were introduced with what is known as the *Codice Rocco* (the Rocco Code) on July 1, 1931, when Italy was still governed by a fascist regime, and are still in force. They are divided into detentive and non-detentive measures (art. 215 of the Italian penal code).

---

[54] Gehlen, A. (1983). Philosophische, Anthropologie und Handlungslehr. Klostermann GmbH.

[55] Lorenz, K. (1966). On Aggression (So-called evil, Toward a Natural History of Aggression). Methuen Publishing.

[56] Ceretti, A., Cornelli, R. (2013). Oltre la paura. Cinque riflessioni su criminalità, società e politica. Feltrinelli.

The detentive measures are divided into *non-psychiatric*, where the person is sent to an agricultural penal colony, a form of open prison, or a penal workshop and if under-age, to a reform school, and *psychiatric*, where the patient with partial mental infirmity is sent to a *Casa di cura e custodia*,[57] and the patient who has been assessed as being totally infirm of mind was previously sent to the FPH, now goes to the REMS. The non-detentive measures include parole, ban on residence in one or more localities, ban on entering pubs or places where alcohol is sold, expulsion from the country (for foreigners without an Italian passport).

Davide also expressed an opinion on following the treatment. "Two pills of Olanzapine a day, one at eight in the morning and one at eight in the evening, I don't know what it does but I do know what it doesn't do, compared with other much less pleasant psychopharmacological drugs. When I take it, I can play music, I can study, the quality of my life is much better than that of lots of people on the other side of these bars. Before I took Olanzapine [...] I was distressed, I was, and the therapy didn't help, in fact, maybe it made things worse because a paranoid who is weakened by Haldol, a paranoid who feels like a herbivore weakened by Haldol surrounded by carnivores becomes even more dangerous because he feels weak. When you feel strong, the paranoia recedes, you've got more space around you, you can breathe better. When you feel weak, the fact of being paranoid and feeling weak, [...] but then I got Doctor P., my benefactor, who prescribed Zyprexa (Olanzapine) in 1998 and Leponex in 1997 (which made the situation better but not completely). But Zyprexa, that's a whole different ball game. If they told me, "You have to take Zyprexa for the rest of your life", No problem. I take my pills in the morning, I put them on my bedside table at night and I take them without anyone having to check on me because they don't bother me at all. If this is the price to pay for being paranoid, two 10 milligram pills of Zyprexa a day, I'm fine with it!"

This acceptance of a psychopharmacological therapy is most unusual in a psychotic as they are generally averse to taking pharmaceutical drugs. Davide's lucidity and awareness of the importance of the treatment could

[57] Casa di cura e custodia: a place of detention, combining treatment and confinement. The mentally infirm, alcoholics and deaf-mutes convicted of a crime are sent to these institutions, as are persons who committed crimes while under the influence of drink or drugs. The mental disturbances cannot be transitory in nature.

be a further element that supports a diagnosis of paranoia rather than paranoid schizophrenia, as usually patients with this latter disorder consider pharmacological treatment as *poison*.

Once taking Olanzapine, Davide's quality of life became acceptable, he played the guitar, joined the FPH theater group led by Monica Franzoni. It was good to see that he found these activities therapeutic in themselves: "You could say that paranoia is an exasperation of opinion; music isn't an opinion, it's a system" and speaking of how actors and musicians work, he says, "Remember that song, the one by Fabri Fibra, "The more you dream, the less you do, the more you do, the less you dream"? Therefore, if you do things as they have to be done or should be done, or if you try to improve them, you dream less and have fewer opinions."

Davide's narrative provided much food for thought: on paranoia, its clinical and nosographic implications; on paranoia and the passage to the act; the subjective and objective dimensions of the patient and the psychiatrist; fear and social dangerousness seen from the point of view of the individual and from that of society, anti-psychotic drugs and treatment.

One element united them all, the subject-Other relationship. Throughout the interview, Davide defined himself as paranoid in relation to the other inmates, doctors, wardens, society, Caterina and I who listened to him. Paranoid, a person who felt the only way out of a given situation was to commit a crime, constantly searching for the objective *perceptum* in relation to his extreme subjectivity, his way of perceiving. A person who could be seen as being dangerous.

The question remains, who is Davide? What is the truth about his personality? Can his crime be completely explained by his paranoia? What does the future hold for him?

Postscript

I found an answer, or at least part of an answer, to that question in November 2023, as I was able to trace Davide to a Casa Alloggio[58] in Reggio Emilia. We had a long talk and, like Fausto, he was happy to share

[58] A "*Casa alloggio*" is a family-style residence with a medium level of protection for adults with a psychic disorder who are moderately autonomous, have sufficient psychosocial capabilities and don't require 24/7 health support.

his impressions and thoughts of how life had treated him since the closure of the FPH, which I have recorded below.

I still haven't made up my mind if a person who is mentally infirm is sick in his mind or has a sick mind.

I'm fine now. Each morning at 9, I see the psychotherapist, I like him and get on really well with him, I'm riding the crest of this wave. This community where I am now, it's a good place; they call it a *Casa alloggio*. That said, the FPH wasn't hell on earth. After I committed that crime, I was sent to an FPH, then to a community in Romagna for seven years, after which I came back to the Reggio Emilia FPH until it was closed. Then I went to a REMS and now, here I am in the *Casa alloggio*.

If I think back on my own history, I have to put in a good word for the FPH, because in that structure you weren't allowed to behave badly. If you let a person behave badly, they will. This is what happens in the REMS, in the communities. Why? Because there is more personal liberty, more everything. I missed the prison-type structure of the FPH when I saw people behaving badly. There were regulations on how to behave, just a minimum, but you respected that. In the communities, the REMS and other more easy-going structures, this code of behaviour doesn't exist and people let fly. Then they have to go into care for a couple of months. Just a thought from an old farmworker from Emilia who has been around.

While I was in the REMS, I attended a theatrical lab, there was a lot of work in that, and I played Macbeth with a Modenese accent. Where I am now, I can do lots of things, I've got a computer in my room, I've got a smart phone, my life is more intense. I can't complain. I even feel good about myself: I continue to study the guitar; I study it with real passion because I love playing it. Every afternoon I study for an hour, sometimes an hour and a half. It does me good, it helps me keep my mind in order because you don't play a guitar with opinions, music isn't an opinion, if you want a certain note you have to put your fingers in a certain way. I find it therapeutic. It's as important to me as the psychotherapist is, I can't do without either. I have a psychiatrist in Sassuolo I see fairly regularly. Every two weeks I go to the Mental Health Center for a Clozapine jab, that drug saved my life. My quality of life was awful before I started taking it; I was full of anti-psychotics and felt bad, I kept changing them hoping to feel better but it didn't happen. Nothing worked. Then a psychiatrist made me try Clozapine and things got better. I was taking two tablets a day but now I get a depot injection every two weeks.

There's one thing I'm proud of: since I've been in the system, I've never said that I'm not mentally ill, but at the same time I've never used this as an excuse. However, if you say I'm mentally ill, you've got to give me some leeway.

When I was young, I gave up reading, then I started again when I was in the FPH. Now I reckon I've read at least a thousand books. There's a little library here, and I made good use of it. Now I order books on Amazon. I buy titles that tickle my curiosity, then if I find references in a book to other books, then I buy those too until I've read everything there is to read on the subject.

What with music and books, I'm satisfied with where I am. They've improved the quality of my life. I can't imagine myself without music and books. After the FPH my life has improved from a practical point of view. I have a room of my own, the only drawback is that it faces north and before the heating gets turned on it's like a refrigerator. But the house is nice, I've never lived in a house as nice as this. Just look at the sky. OK, you could see the sky from the FPH too, but you saw it framed by bars. In the FPH I was in the Centauro ward where they put people who'd committed violent crimes; I wanted to play cards with the others but it just wasn't on, it was better to keep myself to myself. I studied the guitar and read books. I started to do theater there with Monica, the woman in charge of the theater group. I've kept up with her, we exchange cards at Christmas and Easter.

I listened to music and I still do. I have my favourite singers, I could do concerts too, but, although maybe I don't look it, I'm really shy. I can't play in public. I study for myself. Performing to show off what I can do isn't for me. I prefer to wash the plates. Sure, it depends on how many plates and how dirty they are, but here in the *Casa* there are only nine of us. Actually, at the moment there are only eight as one has been hospitalized. It could happen to me too, fortunately I've never been hospitalized in these years but I'm not sure about anything and above all I'm not sure of myself because it doesn't take much to lose it. I don't want to be sure of myself. When you are sure of yourself you make huge mistakes, you feel full of yourself. I prefer to be as I am.

I'm 64 years old. I've got a story to tell about my relationship with alcohol. I always say that I'm like Obelisk and the magic potion. I started drinking wine when I was three years old. I come from a family of farm-workers in Emilia, there was always a bottle of Lambrusco on the table. By the time I was ten I was drinking like a trooper and didn't know it. I only realised at sixty that before my time in the FPH I was always drunk. There's that song by Fabrizio De André, *Amico fragile* (The fragile friend) that describes my life perfectly and closes with the verse "I was much drunker than you". This is it:

> To reach that place called 'till we meet again'
> And it would never have crossed my mind
> That I was much drunker than you
> So very much drunker than you.

This is my song. I realize now that I've drunk my life away. It's like cigarettes, the first ones you smoke make you look cool, you get a taste for them and they make you feel good. Then you get to a certain point when you keep smoking to keep up the intoxication. I gave them up at 43, but I'd been smoking since I was thirteen. It was during that hot summer, the summer of 2003. I was in therapy. They told me to celebrate each time I left the clinic and I decided that I'd buy two packets of cigarettes to celebrate. One evening while I was smoking I took up the diary where I wrote down my thoughts. I thought, "What do I want?" I wrote, "Love, wealth and dreams". I asked myself: "Do I really care about myself"? That very night I smoked the last cigarette. The next day there was the packet lying open with the lighter next to it. I was in my cell and I looked at them without touching them. Stalemate. And that was how I spent the day, in a stalemate. That evening I looked at the books on the table beside my bed that I'd taken out of the library. I picked up one, it was the *Conscience of Zeno* by Italo Svevo. There is this passage in the book where the main character talks about his relationship with tobacco and says, "I lit my last cigarette". I stopped reading, put down the book, put out the light, fell asleep and never touched another cigarette. Zeno was 40 years old when he wrote that book; I was 43. It was a miracle. Miracles do happen.

I enjoy everything, everything in life. I enjoy experimenting. When I was in the FPH, I participated in weekly meetings with don Daniele when we read and discussed the readings of that Sunday's Mass. It was an opportunity to ask questions, discuss, share thoughts. I'm a believer but I allow myself doubts, I'm a follower of Socrates, and I continuously repeat to myself, "I know I don't know". Sometimes during our meetings I'd ask difficult questions and don Daniele, faced with these complicated issues would look at the floor for a bit, and then would say, "We're all poor in spirit". It's true, we're all poor in spirit. But the Bible says that the poor in spirit are better off than anyone else because they have a bigger world in the sense that they lead a wonderful life.

In the REMS my life changed a lot compared to what it was in the FPH. There were lots of stimulus and my quality of life improved. I did lots of things, including theater that I enjoy. I played Macbeth. Now here in the *Casa Alloggio*, if I want to go out, I tell the staff and out I go, I can talk to friends, use my phone, I can talk to whomever I want. In the FPH I was only allowed one telephone call per week to one of the two numbers they permitted me to call. There I didn't have e-mail. Now I don't write much, but I have had periods of continuous contacts. All I had to do was turn on the computer, think of a person and write to them. I've never had a computer before. It's a marvelous world.

I don't allow myself to imagine a future, I don't want to do that because my imagination has caused me a lot of grief. I've put my creativity to one side. Artists use very little imagination; they rely on technique. I think of Bach. No, I've closed with imagination. Now I take what's there when it's there.

Fiorenzo: Impulsiveness and Cocaine

From Playing Calcio Storico *to Prison*

I was a *calciante*, a player in the historical Florentine game known as *Calcio Storico* that takes place every year in Florence. It's a sort of cross between football and rugby, a really violent form of rugby. They say it's the most violent sport in the world. They used to play it in the squares in

Florence, I've played in the Boboli gardens and in piazza Riccardo in San Frediano. These days it's only played in Piazza Santa Croce, right in the heart of the city. I worked as a bouncer, because the *Calcio Storico* is great for finding work as a bodyguard. The players that throw real punches, they end up as bodyguards, working in the discotheques. It's like a shop window for certain jobs.

It's called *Calcio Storico*, or *Florentine kick game*, or *Calcio in Livrea* (Football in Livery). It's been played since the 1500s. In the beginning it was played by the Florentine nobility, including two who became popes. During one game, one of the players drew out a dagger and knifed another player in the leg. Then it became the game of the Florentine militia and finally it was played by the young men of the four Florentine districts: Piazza Santa Croce, San Frediano, Piazza Santa Maria Novella and the greens of San Giovanni, Piazza del Duomo. It's a masculine sport, I'd say. No doubt about that. I was sent to prison for the first time when I was twenty, for getting into a brawl. I did a week and they threw me out. I was a troublemaker because when I was a kid the older boys picked on me and beat me up. In those days I lived near the prison, "delle Murate", there were Sicilians, Calabrians, all borderline; they would beat up us kids, and we played football in a tiny garden, with dog turds all over the place and these guys were really violent. We were scared. I went back and beat them all up. All of them, every last one of them, all, all, all of them. I bust them all and then it started, the prison grind.

Doctor, I Hear Voices

It all started with a brawl when I was twenty, I did a week, then they took me to court, but let me go because I didn't have a record. Then I got sent back five or six times for grievous bodily harm. Then I beat up this guy, another bouncer. There was a war among the bouncers and I punched this guy, broke the bridge of his nose, his cheekbones, smashed his jaw in five places; he was semi-conscious for a week. They gave me eight years and two months. I went in, I'd used up a pardon before and this time I ended up with ten years. I lost it and started fighting with the guards; they beat me up and I cleaned up my act. A month later I beat them up.

But there was a precedent. You want to know how come I ended up in the FPH? It all began with a bit of advice my lawyer gave me. He said, "Fiorenzo, we need to get you acquitted, we need to say you're unfit to plead, diminished responsibility." "But how do I do that, sir?". "You have to say you hear voices." "Voices?". I couldn't figure this out. What was he talking about? Well, he explained everything. Smells, sounds, visions, the lot. I was in prison in Prato. I told the psychiatrist, "Doctor, I hear voices". After a while of me telling him about the voices he said, "Look, I'm not stupid, come off it, you don't hear any voices. You're as fit as a fiddle. You want to go to a lunatic asylum? I'll send you there for a month under observation so you can see for yourself what it's like, if you really want to go. But don't say I didn't warn you". Me, "Yeah, yeah, send me there!".

They Killed Me, Killed Me, Killed Me

They sent me to Montelupo Fiorentino in 1996 and there I told the doctors what the lawyer had told me to say. "I hear voices, I smell the smells of my home" and all the other things my lawyer had taught me.

They started jabbing me, and after twenty days I yelled, "I'm fine, I'm fine, there's nothing wrong with me! The lawyer told me to say those things, send me back to prison!". And they did, right away. But that was a terrible experience I had in the FPH and each time I got into trouble in prison they sent me back there for a month in observation. I must have been there at least fifteen times. It was a really bad place then, now it's a bit better.

At the beginning I beat up the guards. I got kicked in the teeth, clubbed with truncheons, they were really violent, violent with a capital V, they jabbed me full of stuff, slammed me onto restraint beds, I suffered a lot. There was this superintendent, C., she was a beast, bad through and through, and she had it in for me. They played a trick on me. I had to take 50 drops of Minias. They sent me this nurse with a glass full of Entumin; I didn't think anything of it and drank it all down in one gulp. I almost lost consciousness … it's a really strong neuroleptic, but strong!!! The guards came along and tied me onto the restraint bed, they gave me two shots of Entumin a day, two 100 mg shots of Haldol every ten days and two of Clopixol. After fifteen days, there I was, on the restraint bed, and Ignazio Marino[59] came in, he was a Senator then, and I couldn't even speak. They had even given me benzodiazepine, a powerful narcotic. I wanted to talk to him, but I couldn't! And Ignazio Marino said, "Look at the state this man is in! What in the world have you done to him?". The next day they freed me. I got off the bed and collapsed, I had no strength at all. I've put on weight, I used to weigh 90 kg and at the end I weighed 120 after a year of those injections.

They killed me, killed, killed, killed me. Thank God I'm strong and even if I'm getting on in years now, I'll be 52 in May .... I was in the maximum-security jail in Spoleto and they refused to send me to the penal section. "Why don't you want to send me to the penal section? I've already done fifteen years..." Well, finally I set fire to three cells and they sent me back here as mentally handicapped under the terms of article 111. Now, if they hold you under the terms of 111 and you want to go back to prison, all you need is a psychiatrist to say you are sane of mind, not like the 148, there you need a judge to revoke the order.

Now things are going fine. They let me out ninety days ahead of schedule for perfect conduct, best behaviour, the first time in twenty years; they gave me a two-hour license to go visit my mother who's very sick. Now I hope things will start moving; I'll ask to get assigned to the Social Services. I hope this will be the end of the matter because I can't take anymore. I'm worn out.

For Three Months Now, I Run an Hour Each Day

I run every morning for an hour. I've already lost about 15 kg, now I weigh 105, from 120. I've been doing this for the last three months now; it's not long. And six months ago they stopped the depot. I'd been on that for three years! They've destroyed me! They've really destroyed me! They've ruined my strength. My legs hurt, I couldn't walk, not even a couple of steps and now my knee hurts when I run. I had a bad accident, I can do

[59] Ignazio Marino, Senator of the Italian Republic, chaired a Parliamentary Commission investigating the FPH which contributed to their closure.

an hour no problem, and a quarter of an hour of stretching. Then I do some exercises in my cell, pull-ups on the bed, vertical push-ups, I'm getting my strength back, I've got 20% more strength now.

I'm friends with P., he's a 148, he's very intelligent and sensitive and he's the only normal guy in the section.

I'm suffering, suffering, suffering, suffering, suffering. I'm alone and the afternoons are endless. Hardly any films, I really like *The Gladiator* but I've seen it hundreds of times. The first time I saw it I cried. Massimo Meridio. Russell Crowe is great.

I didn't really get into the leading character… but the character got to me. A splendid film. *The Green Mile* was good, so was *The Shawshank Redemption, The Godfather, Once upon a time in America*, Al Pacino and Scarface… all a bit violent!

Robert De Niro now, I saw the trailer of a film with him as a boxer, just him! He's 200 years old! When he was young and wild, OK, but now…

Getting back to this place… do I feel I've been cured of the impulsiveness and the anger? I feel more mature. Mature. Nobody helped me in this.

I always use the '*tu*' form with the guards, my dad said to use the '*lei*' form and '*voi*' when talking to older people. My dad was a gentleman, he was a tailor. He died of lung cancer when he was fifty.

I lost a brother to lung cancer two years ago. I've a CT scan at the end of the month. If it's OK I'll cut down a packet a day right away. I smoke 35 cigarettes a day and it's too much.

I was saying that I matured all by myself. I've never got on with the guards, but Fiorenzo is a gentleman. And if I say it myself, then it's true. He's not violent, he's well behaved, always uses the '*lei*' form. They have said to me, "Fiorenzo, you have changed radically". I get on with the guards. I want it to be that way. At the beginning I was aggressive with them… but they were aggressive with me too. They hurt my head. They hammered me, burnt my wrists, burnt me with their cigarettes, they gave me 400 cc of methadone to sedate me, I went into a state of coma vigil, pneumonia, pericarditis and coma vigil. I was at death's door lots of times, once they got me just in time, in Parma, I was dying. They kicked me in the teeth, I saw my blood flowing but I couldn't get my mind round what was happening. It was choking me, I was losing it… I couldn't understand why I was feeling so bad. Why, why was I feeling so bad? They just got me in time, there in the prison in Parma. I was a hair's breadth from death. I must have a little angel looking after me, who knows?

I Really Look Forward to the Visits

It was a terrible moment, really traumatic. My Dad died in 1979.

My mum, she's a saint, she worked a lot, and she brought us all up on her own. She was an excellent cook.

She never came to see me play in the matches, no, no. She has a strong character, she's robust, but now she's very ill. I'm scared I'll lose her. I lost a brother, I've a pain here, in my heart. He died, suffocated by his own blood. He had lung cancer.

I've been able to see them, my mum and my brother, over the past years… yes, they let me have two years for incompatibility, I was out for two years.

I've got a sister, she's the oldest of the family. She's a manager. Then there's R. He was having an operation and they messed it up. He went into septicemia and they almost lost him. My sister's brother-in-law is a very good surgeon and he saved him. You can die of septicemia, eh! He manages a day up, then he has to go back to bed. He's got a daughter, she's in the fifth year of language school, it's a private school and costs a fortune. I don't get her to come here. I go to them on Saturdays.

I really enjoy the visits. I love my family, and after Francesco died we've become even closer than before.

We can have a visit from family once a month, but we don't have much money and I don't want them to have to spend money; mum's OK with that, the important thing is that they are well.

I do look forward to their visit. It's a way of getting in touch with the world outside. Now they've granted me early release, a whole ninety days, I've got to set the date to go home to my mamma.

These Aren't Hospitals, They Are Criminal Lunatic Asylums

I've got a new psychiatrist now, G. I get on fairly well with him.

I knew him by sight, before I had a psychiatrist. She was very good. I call her every day to come visit me, but I don't know why... I guess she's very busy.

Is this place useful? Who knows? Now I'm taking Lithium Salts and Tolep. I know they are toxic but I just get a minimum dose. They don't do anything for me, I've had them before, but as we say in Florence, they are *birbonate,* a joke. I read the leaflet on Lithium Salts, they say you should do the lithaemia to test the level of lithium because it's toxic and they don't know exactly what it does to your mind? It's supposed to be a stabilizer, but who knows? At the physiological level... science doesn't know. Are my moods more stable? A little. I don't feel anything.

But I do feel less sedated than before... and I don't have the urge to beat someone up. I've finished with violence. OK, let's put it this way; if someone comes along and punches me, I'll defend myself, I'm not dumb. I can still hold my own!

However, in three months I've lost half of the weight I put on. I was 120 kg, now I'm 105. That's 15 kg. I've got to get back to 90 kg. A year's running, that's what it'll take. It's just that this knee really gives me gyp.

These aren't Forensic Hospitals, they are Lunatic Asylums for Criminals. A euphemism isn't going to change the reality. What's this place got in common with a hospital? You can see for yourself. These are cells. Barcellona Pozzo di Gotto in Sicily is much better; I was there in 2006. They've got a garden, a bar, they show films, the sections were open. The only thing was, I was a long way from home, the family couldn't come to visit. I was going out with this girl, she came to see me once a month, but my family no. We aren't very well off, and just now, well, we're all struggling to make ends meet, aren't we?

I've done more than forty stretches in prison, a long career you could say, all because I'm impulsive. I'm very reactive. Like I said, my first experience in the Forensic Hospitals was in '96 because of the bad advice I got from my lawyer. I said I had symptoms that I didn't have. I've never heard voices in my life. I thought the lawyer was giving me a good tip...

After that, every time I had an episode they shoved me into observation for a month.

When you've been there once, it's a precedent, there's no end to it.

"Ah, he's been in the loony bin, he's unmanageable so send him back there. They'll sedate him."

Have I ever been ill in my head? No, only when they injected me with all that stuff. I've done lots of tests that show there's nothing wrong with my head.

That impulsive streak in my character, is linked to the circumstances, to the people I hung out with … the group of football players… Something I've learned or something I've thought out for myself? I was born into that environment with all those big guys, I was fascinated. All of us who lived in the historical centre of Florence, it was like the Palio di Siena, they do it with horses, but I'm against that. I'm for the animals; when you're with humans you know what you're doing; like with the bulls in Spain, I'd avoid that. Playing football was a way of letting off steam.

Then I did it for the women, women liked the strongest guys, there was plenty of competition.

"Fiorenzo, you're so impulsive!"

There are some really sick people here. I know you can't cure schizophrenia. Sure, there are depots, but you don't get better. When you go into psychosis, your mind doesn't work anymore. These people are delirious, if you say hello to them, they reply "uaaaagh". They are really sick. There's no cure for schizophrenia.

In my experience crimes aren't linked to an illness but rather to a way of being….

I've spent quite some time in Rehab and a professor there said to me, "Fiorenzo, you're impulsive and reactive by nature, and you like cocaine."

It's true, I liked cocaine, less now than before: when I went to the disco at the weekends, I'd take 3–4 grams.

That means putting yourself in a state in which you are a danger to others.

Now, to be honest, I don't feel I'm dangerous anymore. But what I did… I think I'm the only inmate who's done 25 years for punching. I've never killed anyone, never sold drugs, never stole anything. All I ever did was GBH, GBH, GBH, GBH, GBH.

The future is hard for everyone. There are young engineers who go to work in the fields, who can't find work at all, who emigrate to the States to work because there's nothing here. Life's tough for everyone. I've got a pension, 80% of the full pension. I get 180 euro, and I've got a job, I think it'll still be there. Riding therapy, that's my job. I help children with problems, autism, Down syndrome, other pathologies, to ride a horse. I take them around the circuit, and they change as you take them round slowly, I like doing something useful.

Reflections on Fiorenzo's Story

Fiorenzo is in his fifties, physically robust, with a pleasant face. We have an appointment in the school-room, we sit at the desks and listen to him as if he were a professor giving a lecture. He's wearing an old coat with a fur collar.

His story is complicated. He played the Florentine game of *Calcio Storico*,[60] a very violent form of rugby, "the most violent sport in the world" that threw him into the spotlight in Florence. It was a sort of shop window for men wanting to become body guards, or looking for a woman ("I did it for the women, women liked strong men, there was competition"). So, he was playing a game in which violence was not only acceptable, it was the rule, a rule that enhanced certain individual characteristics. A similar intermingling between individual factors and a social-sport profile can also be found in other sports, such as boxing, as the American psychiatrist Donald W. Black pointed out in his book "*Bad Boys, Bad Men*".

"Antisocials who become boxers, wrestlers or soldiers are not unheard of, though most lack the discipline or tolerance for regulations that such occupations require. I would not profess to diagnose Mike Tyson with

[60] Bennucci, S., Bini, U., Giovannelli, F. (2012). Il Calcio Fiorentino. EDK Editore.

ASP or any other condition, but his history reveals the aggressive tendencies associated with antisocial personality."[61]

Fiorenzo's story is a long list of spells in prison from the age of twenty, all for GBH; it reflects an impulsive and reactive personality, a childhood he says was tainted by being bullied by bigger boys, but who he paid back in kind, "I went back and beat them all up. All of them, every last one of them, all, all, all of them. I busted them all…". As a young man, the *Calcio Storico* provided him with the perfect context for his impulsivity and inclination to violence, he enjoyed it ("it was a way of letting off steam"). Parallel to his involvement in sports, there is the cocaine. Cocaine is ever present in Fiorenzo's story. His clinical data compare positively to the four criteria of the antisocial personality disorder (ASP) as listed in DSM-5:

1. Disregard for and violation of others rights since age 15, as indicated by one of the seven sub features: failure to obey laws and norms by engaging in behavior which results in criminal arrest, or would warrant criminal arrest; lying, deception, and manipulation, for profit or self-amusement; impulsive behavior; irritability and aggression, manifested as frequently assaults others, or engages in fighting; blatantly disregards safety of self and others; a pattern of irresponsibility and lack of remorse for actions.
2. The person is at least age 18;
3. Conduct disorder was present by history before age 15;
4. The antisocial behavior does not occur in the context of schizophrenia or bipolar disorder (American Psychiatric Association, 2013).[62]

Fiorenzo appears to tick all the boxes for Antisocial Personality Disorder. Under point A, DSM-5 cites impulsive behaviour as an indication of ASP, but what exactly does impulsive behaviour entail? Fiorenzo says he did "more than forty stretches in prison, a long career you could say, all because I'm impulsive". What is the link between impulsiveness and crime?

---

[61] Black, D.W. (2013). Bad Boys, Bad Men: Confronting Antisocial Personality Disorder (Sociopathy) Revised Edition. Oxford University Press.

[62] *Antisocial Personality Disorder* in American Psychiatric Association. (2013). *Diagnostic and Statistical Manual of Mental Disorders* (5th ed.). American Psychiatric Publishing, pp. 659–663.

In psychology, impulsivity or impulsiveness (from the Latin impellere, to push before) is a tendency to act on a whim, displaying behavior characterized by little or no forethought, reflection, or consideration of the consequences.[63] Impulsive actions are typically "poorly conceived, prematurely expressed, unduly risky, or inappropriate to the situation that often result in undesirable consequences,"[64] which imperil long-term goals and strategies for success.[65] Impulsivity can be classified as a multifactorial construct.[66]

According to the Swiss psychiatrist Eugen Bleuler, impulsivity as a symptom is not well-defined but rather is a manner in which pathological actions are manifested. Some impulsive actions are automatic, others are dominated by the affective framework, or the release of emotive tension. Impulsive actions are egosyntonic because the intentionality outweighs the forced aspect. The actions are gratifying because they vent bad feelings, frustration, and depression, even if this gratification, which is usually sexual or aggressive in nature, is pathologically twisted and reveals the incapacity of the person to deal with these feelings.[67]

Fiorenzo landed in prison for GBH, and even inside, he continued to act on impulse, attacking the prison guards with the result that they fought back and Fiorenzo, alone against many, certainly got the worst of it. In fact, his impulsive behaviour turns against him and in the end results in what amounts to self-harm. Daphne Simeon and Armando R. Favazza describe such behaviour as deliberately inflicting physical pain on one's own body without any intention that such an act should lead to death. In this definition the term *deliberately* implicates a conscious intent rather than a motivation impelled by the subconscious. These authors

---

[63] American Psychological Association. (2007). *APA Dictionary of Psychology*. American Psychological Association (APA).

[64] Daruna, J. H., & Barnes, P. A. (1993). A neurodevelopmental view of impulsivity. *The Impulsive Client: Theory, Research, and Treatment.*, 23–37. https://doi.org/10.1037/10500-002

[65] Madden, Gregory J., Johnson, Patrick S. (2010). *"A Delay-Discounting Primer"*. In Madden, Gregory Jude; Bickel, Warren K. (eds.). *Impulsivity: The Behavioral and Neurological Science of Discounting*. Washington, DC: American Psychological Association. pp. 11–37. ISBN 978-1-4338-0477-9.

[66] Evenden, J. L. (1999). Varieties of impulsivity. *Psychopharmacology*, *146*(4), 348–361. https://doi.org/10.1007/pl00005481

[67] Bleuler, E. (1924). Textbook of Psychiatry. Macmillan.

also note that certain individuals impulsively inflict self-injury only a few times in their lives, while others do so regularly. The terms *episodic* and *repetitive* can be used to differentiate these two types of patients. In repetitive patients, this self-injurious behavior becomes a structural and predominant preoccupation, it is like an addiction and is incorporated into the sense of the individual's sense of identity.[68]

Violent, hot-headed, quarrelsome, provocative, impulsive; all these adjectives describe Fiorenzo. He continuously aggravates the Other (in the sense of the Lacanian Other-of language or Other of relationships), the bouncers, guards, *enemies* of all types and kinds so as to provoke fights and brawls in which he gets hurt as much as he hurts his opponents. This is the identity that Fiorenzo constructed for himself in Florence, in prison and in the FPH where he was sent for periods of observation or treatment. In the FPH in fact, his impulsivity is treated with anti-psychotic drugs. His account of when he was sedated is particularly clear and detailed, "They sent me this nurse with a glass full of Entumin; I didn't suspect anything and drank it all down in one gulp. I almost lost consciousness … it's a really strong neuroleptic, but strong!!!. The guards came along and tied me onto the restraint bed, they gave me two shots of Entumin a day, two 100 mg shots of Haldol every ten days and two of Clopixol" to the point that when the Head of the Parliamentary Commission came to visit the FPH, "there I was, on the restraint bed, and Ignazio Marino[69] came in, he was a Senator then, and I couldn't even speak. They had even given me benzodiazepine, a powerful narcotic. I wanted to talk to him, but I couldn't! And Ignazio Marino said, "Look at the state this man is in! What in the world have you done to him?".

Fiorenzo's impulsive self-injurious behavior can be interpreted on the basis of these criteria proposed by Simeon and Favazza:[70]

---

[68] Simeon, D., & Favazza, A. R. (2001). Self-injurious behaviors: Phenomenology and assessment. In D. Simeon & E. Hollander (Eds.), *Self-injurious behaviors: Assessment and treatment* (pp. 1–28). American Psychiatric Publishing, Inc.

[69] Ignazio Marino, Senator of the Italian Republic, chaired a Parliamentary Commission investigating the FPH which contributed to their closure.

[70] Simeon, D., & Favazza, A. R. (2001). Self-injurious behaviors: Phenomenology and assessment. In D. Simeon & E. Hollander (Eds.), *Self-injurious behaviors: Assessment and treatment* (pp. 1–28). American Psychiatric Publishing, Inc.

- The need to hurt himself physically;
- Recurring failure to resist the impulse to hurt himself to the extent of procuring the destruction or alteration of body tissues;
- An increased feeling of tension immediately prior to self-injury;
- A sense of gratification or relief when committing self-injury;
- The act of self-injury is not associated with suicidal intentions or psychosis, transsexuality, mental deficiency or developmental disorder.

In an article published in 1976, Matti Virkkunen, professor of Forensic Psychiatry at the Helsinki University Central Hospital (HUCH), emphasized how self-mutilation is strongly associated with ASP and other personality disorders, with aggressivity, and violence and hypothesized that the dearth of stimuli in the prison environment could act as a catalyst for self-injury in sensation-seeking sociopaths. Moreover, the self-injury may be inflicted at the time of imprisonment[71] or, as some other authors sustain, may precede it by a long period.[72,73] In an article written in 1997, Carl Fulwiler and colleagues state that over 50% of the sample in their study declared that the purpose of self-mutilation was to relieve anxiety or tension.[74]

In addition to his accounts of his impulsive and violent behavior, Fiorenzo also talks about his use, abuse, of drugs. In an article written in 2007, Samuel Chamberlain and Barbara Sahakian noted that addiction to cocaine is associated with an increase in impulsivity.[75] At the same time, impulsivity could be a premorbid trait that increases vulnerability to cocaine addiction, and both the addition and the impulsive behavior

[71] Virkkunen, M. (1976). Self-mutilation in antisocial personality (disorder). *Acta Psychiatrica Scandinavica, 54*(5), 347–352. https://doi.org/10.1111/j.1600-0447.1976.tb00130.x

[72] Paulino, A.F.G., Krolikowski, F.J. (1995). Insertion of Foreign Bodies into the Abdominal Cavity. *American Journal of Forensic Medicine and Pathology, 16*, 48–50.

[73] Rada, R.T., James, W. (1982). Urethral Insertion of Foreign Bodies: a Report of Contagious Self-Mutilation in a Maximum Security Hospital. *Archives of General Psychiatry, 39*, 423–429.

[74] Fulwiler, C., Forbes, C., Santangelo, S.L., Folstein, M. (1997). Self-Mutilation and Suicide Attempt: Distinguishing Features in Prisoners. *Journal of the American Academy of Psychiatry and the Law, 25*, 69–77.

[75] Chamberlain, S., & Sahakian, B.J. (2007). The neuropsychiatry of impulsivity. *Current Opinion in Psychiatry, 20*, 255–261.

are regulated by the cortico-striatal network:[76] addiction theories maintain that impulsivity and substance abuse are caused by inadequate communication between the behavioral control centers in the prefrontal cortex and the motivational subcortical (striatal) circuits.[77] A group of Spanish authors, in *Clinical Differences Between Cocaine-Dependent Patients With and Without Antisocial Personality Disorder*, maintained that "cocaine addiction is one of the factors that is most strongly associated in antisocial personality disorder", and "cocaine users frequently experience paranoid delirium with visual and auditive hallucinations, symptoms that correlate with an erroneous interpretation of the surrounding stimuli and a perception of the environment as being hostile, which easily results in them manifesting aggressive or antisocial behavior." They also say that violent people may take drugs like cocaine to reduce their anxiety and inhibitions regarding breaking the law and causing harm to others. The authors noted that their sample of cocaine addicts with antisocial personality disorder were tendentially young, single, with a low level of education, unemployed and with a higher probability of being imprisoned compared to the control group of cocaine addicts who were not suffering from antisocial personality disorder.[78]

Another group of Spanish researchers led by Natalia Albein-Urios, working on the correlates of neuroimaging in drug addicts, found that in terms of cognitive-affective functioning, cocaine dependent patients with comorbid personality disorders, compared to cocaine dependent patients without comorbid personality disorders, showed higher levels of impulsivity fuelled by negative emotions (negative urgency), borderline beliefs associated with personality pathologies, a lower capacity for cognitive control and reduced gray temporal pole matter in the regions of the brain

---

[76] Cunningham, K. A., & Anastasio, N. C. (2014). Serotonin at the nexus of impulsivity and cue reactivity in cocaine addiction. *Neuropharmacology, 76*(Part B), 460–478. https://doi.org/10.1016/j.neuropharm.2013.06.030

[77] Bickel, W. K., Miller, M. L., Yi, R., Kowal, B. P., Lindquist, D. M., & Pitcock, J. A. (2007). Behavioral and neuroeconomics of drug addiction: Competing neural systems and temporal discounting processes. *Drug and Alcohol Dependence, 90,* S85–S91. https://doi.org/10.1016/j.drugalcdep.2006.09.016

[78] Comín, M., Redondo, S., Daigre, C., Grau-López, L., Casas, M., & Roncero, C. (2016). Clinical differences between cocaine-dependent patients with and without antisocial personality disorder. *Psychiatry Research, 246*, 587–592. https://doi.org/10.1016/j.psychres.2016.10.083

that are relevant for social-emotional cognition. Given that cocaine addiction and Cluster B personality disorders are associated with dysfunctions in the cerebral regions and connections that support emotional control, the co-occurrence of these two diagnoses could cause more severe deficits in these regions and connections.[79]

This study found that cocaine users with comorbid Cluster B personality disorders show reduced activation of the subgenual anterior cingulate cortex (subgenual ACC) and increased activations of the lateral orbitofrontal cortex and the amygdale during cognitive reappraisal, which is particularly interesting when compared to what Antoine Bechara and colleagues wrote in 1994 on the insensitivity to future consequences of decision making process in individuals with cerebral lesions in the area of the subgenual ACC;[80] in other words, these individuals have a functional deficit in the cerebral regions that support the experiential and learning aspects of negative emotions.

It is interesting to note that in addition to the research on structural cerebral alterations in individuals affected by antisocial personality disorders, groups of researchers are now investigating genes correlated with antisocial behavior. Rautiainen and colleagues conducted a genome-wide association study (GWAS) on 173 Finnish criminal offenders and 3766 controls, which evidenced suggestive associations of two clusters of single-nucleotide polymorphisms at 6p21.2 and at 6p21.32 at the human leukocyte antigen (HLA) region. Two polymorphisms in the genic regions LINC00951 and LRFN2 at 6p21.2 are both expressed in the brain, especially in the frontal cortex, which is intriguing considering the role of the frontal cortex in behavior and the neuroanatomical findings of reduced gray matter volume in antisocial personality disorders.[81]

---

[79] Albein-Urios, N., Martínez-González, J. M., Lozano, Ó., Moreno-López, L., Soriano-Mas, C., & Verdejo-García, A. (2013). Negative urgency, disinhibition and reduced temporal pole gray matter characterize the comorbidity of cocaine dependence and personality disorders. *Drug and Alcohol Dependence, 132*(1–2), 231–237. https://doi.org/10.1016/j.drugalcdep.2013.02.008

[80] Bechara, A., Damásio, A. R., Damásio, H., & Anderson, S. W. (1994). Insensitivity to future consequences following damage to human prefrontal cortex. *Cognition, 50*(1–3), 7–15. https://doi.org/10.1016/0010-0277(94)90018-3

[81] Rautiainen, M., Paunio, T., Repo-Tiihonen, E., Virkkunen, M., Ollila, H., Sulkava, S., Jolanki, O., Palotie, A., & Tiihonen, J. (2016). Genome-wide association study of antisocial personality disorder. *Translational Psychiatry, 6*(9), e883. https://doi.org/10.1038/tp.2016.155

Jari Tiihonen and colleagues, studying two independent cohorts of Finnish prisoners, noted that a monoamine oxidase A (MAOA) low-activity genotype (contributing to low dopamine turnover rate) and the CDH13 gene (coding for neuronal membrane adhesion protein) are associated with extremely violent behavior.[82] Jessica Salvatore and colleagues found a significant correlation between the expression of the gene ABCB1 and addiction to cocaine and alcohol, and a greater correlation between that same gene and the immune pathways and externalising behavior.[83]

However, even these studies on the possible neurobiological alterations in ASP comorbid with cocaine abuse and the findings regarding genetics do not come close to answering the question: where is the evil located? This is an important question that concerns everyone, not only those suffering from a mental illness. Fiorenzo is not suffering from a severe mental disorder that would have fallen into the DSM's Axis 1,[84] his was more a question of character which at a certain point in his life revealed its more pathological aspects, including a dominant impulsivity. His crimes were not linked to delusions or hallucinations that impacted his ability to make sound judgements and understand the consequences of his acts. The question is, to what extent can Fiorenzo be held responsible for the crimes he committed?

In "*What does recent neuroscience tell us about Criminal responsibility*" Uri Maoz and Gideon Yaffe discussed the potential of neuroscientific

[82] Tiihonen, J., Rautiainen, M., Ollila, H., Repo-Tiihonen, E., Virkkunen, M., Palotie, A., Pietiläinen, O., Kristiansson, K., Joukamaa, M., Lauerma, H., Saarela, J., Tyni, S., Vartiainen, H., Paananen, J., Goldman, D., & Paunio, T. (2014). Genetic background of extreme violent behavior. *Molecular Psychiatry, 20*(6), 786–792. https://doi.org/10.1038/mp.2014.130

[83] Salvatore, J. E., Edwards, A. C., McClintick, J. N., Bigdeli, T. B., Adkins, A., Aliev, F., Edenberg, H. J., Foroud, T., Hesselbrock, Kramer, J., Nürnberger, J. I., Schuckit, M. A., Tischfield, J. A., Xuei, X., & Dick, D. M. (2015). Genome-wide association data suggest ABCB1 and immune-related gene sets may be involved in adult antisocial behavior. *Translational Psychiatry, 5*(4), e558. https://doi.org/10.1038/tp.2015.36

[84] DSM-IV used a multi-axial formulation (American Psychiatric Association, 2013b) for psychiatric assessment and organization of biopsychosocial information. There were five different axes: Axis I consisted of mental health and substance use disorders (SUDs); Axis II was reserved for personality disorders and mental retardation; Axis III was used for coding general medical conditions; Axis IV was to note psychosocial and environmental problems (e.g., housing, employment); and Axis V was an assessment of overall functioning known as the GAF. This multi-axial approach was dropped in DSM-5.

experimentation to "illuminate the nature and underlying mechanisms of features that contribute to and constitute criminal responsibility" both in healthy subjects and in those suffering from mental illness, because "Criminal behavior is a product of the interaction between the states and functional dispositions of the brain, on the one hand, and the environment, on the other".[85]

Investigating evil from a scientific standpoint is no easy matter. Indeed, according to Simon Baron-Cohen, the concept of evil is unhelpful and unscientific. In his book entitled "*The science of evil: On empathy and the origins of cruelty*",[86] he proposes using the concept of "empathy erosion" to understand cruelty. In cases where people are treated as inanimate objects, empathy is absent. Indeed, there is little evidence of empathy in Fiorenzo's story, and a quantification of his capacity for empathy and of its level of impairment, along the lines described by Baron-Cohen, could be useful to study its implications for Fiorenzo's crimes and even, possibly, a functional recovery.

In 2005, the United Sections of the Italian Court of Cassation issued a decision regarding serious personality disorders which is of interest to Fiorenzo's case and mental illnesses. It states that

"Personality disorders, such as neurosis and psychopathy, can be considered as acceptable reasons for excluding, or greatly reducing, the legal competence of an individual [...], as long as they are present in such a degree, intensity and gravity as to effectively impact on such competence. Conversely, the other "characterial anomalies" and "emotional and passionate" that in terms of intensity and gravity do not affect the individual's capacity for self-determination, are not considered as having an effect on imputability. There must also be a causative link between the mental disorder and the crime, so that the latter may be considered as being determined by the former."[87]

As mentioned before, Fiorenzo's story is a long list of periods spent in prison, with a first experience in an FPH in 1996 when he told the prison

---

[85] Maoz, U., & Yaffe, G. (2015). What does recent neuroscience tell us about criminal responsibility? *Journal of Law and the Biosciences*, *3*(1), 120–139. https://doi.org/10.1093/jlb/lsv051

[86] Baron-Cohen, S. (2012). *The science of evil: On Empathy and the Origins of Cruelty*.

[87] https://www.altalex.com/documents/news/2006/09/12/i-gravi-disturbi-della-personalita-rientrano-nel-concetto-di-infermita-mentale

psychiatrist he was hearing voices, on the advice of his lawyer who was trying to have him acquitted. This episode became a precedent, and so every time he was involved in a brawl in prison, he was sent to the FPH in observation, or in certain cases, as a mentally handicapped person.

We do not know if Fiorenzo's lawyer attempted to have him acquitted under the terms of the sentence of the Court of Cassation mentioned above. It is interesting to note that with this ruling Italian justice has to a certain extent pathologized crime. However, not all forensic psychiatrists and criminologists were of the opinion that personality disorders can affect the legal competence of a person who has committed a crime and so contribute to the case for an acquittal.

In his book "*La violenza. Dentro di noi, attorno a noi*", Vittorino Andreoli, Italian psychiatrist and author of numerous texts on psychology and psychiatry, spoke of human violence in these terms, "There is a violent io inside me. Usually I carry it about, unaware of its existence, but sometimes it becomes agitated and shakes the statue of my body. It lives like a gentle twin inside me, it is not even able to tear off a yellowing leaf in the autumn. Inside me, there is violence and goodness, destructiveness and love".[88] In an interview on leading Italian daily Corriere della Sera in 2017, speaking of the increase in episodes of violence in the family, he stated, "Today we are living in an increasingly instinctual society, in which taboos no longer exist and there are no longer any inhibitions within the family circle: paradoxically, we are becoming most violent towards the people who love us most. This is because the family, like the school, has lost its connotations of authority, respect, education, cohesion. Even within the home, death has lost its mystery, has become banal as if it were just another illness: an anti-educational equivalence".[89]

As we continue to explore the concept of evil, the issue evolves from "where is it?", to "what is it?". The search for answers to these questions should not be limited to the world of individuals suffering from psychiatric pathologies but also include that of so-called normal people who commit acts of evil.[90]

---

[88] Andreoli, V. (1993). *La Violenza. Dentro di noi, attorno a noi*, Rizzoli. 278.

[89] Andreoli, V. (2017). Famiglia e scuola senza autorità sono percepite come un ostacolo. *Corriere della Sera,* 12 January 2017, 18.

[90] Binik, O. (2020). *The Fascination with Violence in Contemporary Society: When Crime is Sublime.* Palgrave Macmillan.

Giovanni: Megalomaniacal Delirium and the Nato

I Knew the NATO's Monitoring Systems

Now that's a good question! I wonder now, how long has mental illness been around? Because I don't know what mental illness is… it could be a sort of disturbance, that distorts your vision of reality so it isn't in line with the accepted standards. But then you have to see what the media want; the media are the great giants of the world. You need to know all about the media: names, surnames, addresses, fiscal code numbers, their current economic interests and how they shepherd the masses by conditioning them psychologically with their advertising promotions in television commercials or any other form of commercial, so that civil educated people have to use, consume and live to be able to exist in society.

I'm suffering from a grave form of amnesia… when my memories are like a mosaic, with illuminated mnemonic points of my past, enveloped in a great mist, a great confusion of ideas. The doctor says I'm suffering from delusion, that I have a severe paranoid personality disorder and a narcissistic personality disorder as I am subject to grandiose delusions, sometimes borderline, and so my psychiatric condition swings from one pathology to the other. That's what the doctor says.

And what do I say? First of all, you need to start from the psychiatric report that was published on the Turin newspaper, "La Stampa di Torino" under the section "Cronaca di Torino", even before the hearing and I've got something to say about that, about information from the pre-trial hearing being printed before it even took place. Yes, I've got plenty to say about that, plenty. What I say is, I suffer from amnesia, and my amnesia hasn't been caused by a shock, a shock from natural circumstances, it was caused by blunt force or neuro degenerative substances such as Scopolamine, Pentothal…

They accused me of a double murder. I was in Barcelona, Spain when it happened and if there's a magistrate that wants to challenge their majesties the public prosecutor of Turin and the two attorneys who were in Barcelona too. They hypno-induced me with that flying circus that attacked me on July 15, 2004 at 16.30 on the beach at Barceloneta, between the touristic port and the … where there is a big Baywatch type lifeguard tower and lifeguards, I was attacked there and hypno-induced to go to Turin. "You've got to go back to Turin".

I was a physicist/nuclear engineer, I was involved in geo-technology, but I only remembered that three years later, not right away.

I knew some surveillance systems that the countries in NATO use. They use surveillance systems with geo-technology, there's a data processing center with volumetric telecameras, everything that you see in the parallelepiped is to scan [sic] every single room, even the one we're in now. We're in cybernetic technology, we're not in the prehistory of technology anymore. They said to me, "How come you know the name of the company that distributes these technologies?" I worked for that company. They don't show that on television, eh no. They screwed me well and truly, they were good. This went on from 1994 with Turin, and in 2004 they managed to screw me, good and proper. The General Public Prosecutor wanted to speed up the implementation of urbanistic structures and surveillance-safety measures. Helping him to pick up his pen and put his signature to the implementation of structural works… because without his signature the implementation can't go ahead.

I was in prison in Turin, then I was in Saluzzo for nine months, and before that there in a penal section. I wasn't always in the psychiatric section in Turin but I wanted to take a step back doctor. I spent eighteen months in the "Psychiatric Observation" unit in Turin, because I had the Appeal and the Court of Cassation, in Appeal and Court of Cassation it's possible to do a psychiatric review and that's why I spent eighteen months there. Those two big-headed prosecutors in Barcelona, I was there for thirty-two months, thirty-six months and maybe a bit longer because there was an adjacent section that they call "Il Sestante", a penal "pre-section". There's an adjustment of the person's psychiatric condition, the idea being that the person is rehabilitated to live in a different context to the twenty-four-hour surveillance mode, with a bed nailed to the floor and tables fixed to the walls. There used to be regular tables, cupboards… The Centauro wing, which is chaotic due to the inmates' pathologies, is child's play compared to the three years I spent there. Why did I spend three years there? I'm the only person who spent three years there. Why? Why did I have to stay there if they had already decided on the sentence?

And they did everything off their own bat because I hired lawyers then fired them. They assigned me a court-appointed lawyer, who practically gave the closing argument for the prosecution at the final hearing. Finally, those two procurators stood up and said, "No, we're fine with thirty years" because he wanted me to get forty, twenty plus twenty. "We're fine with thirty". And I've plenty to say about that too. Plenty. But going back to your question… I've lost the thread…

How did the mental illness lead to the crime?

I didn't commit any crime. I was in Barcelona, Spain. If there's a magistrate with the strength, the coherency, the social and cultural values to challenge his majesty the General Public Prosecutor of Turin, they could demonstrate that and have me released. This was a deliberate and well-orchestrated decision, right from 1994. Like I said before, that Prosecutor wanted to speed up the implementation of those works in a way that I prefer to keep to myself. Then in 2004, then the ordeal began. The mishap in 1994 and the ordeal in 2004. When I arrived here, I met good people with humanitarian values, people who take an interest in you, who look after you and take care of you.

They Decided I Live a Delusion

My day starts at eight in the morning when they wake me up for therapy. I live in a state of mental confusion until about ten o' clock, but at nine I work as a barber, just a small job I found here to have a minimum subsidy. Before I ended up here in the FPH I was well off economically. When they arrested me, I endured six years of censure, indignity; I was treated badly, bullied, subjected to all sorts of harassment, and provoked; they even made me wrestle. They never beat me up directly but they did when I was asleep, and I woke up covered in bruises and contusions. When I was in the psychiatric ward in Turin from 2004 to 2007, if you had a headache and needed a pill, you had to bang the windows and slam the doors or they wouldn't give you a pill for the headache because whatever I said, it wasn't true. Then they decided that I *live a delusion.* After six years of prison, after what was a really appalling and shocking period, they decided that I have delusions and a mental illness. I became a 148 which is the worst thing that can happen to you because you aren't, say, "suitable for prison life" because you are mentally disturbed and at the same time they can't release you because you have been sentenced to imprisonment. So they bundle you off to the FPH, this rubbish dump. The institutions don't do what they should with the Communities, because the Communities aren't genuine rehabilitation structures for re-inserting people into society. The Community is only a transitional phase between here and the outside, here and freedom. But to get back to the FPH… a typical day… we were saying… the afternoon… when I can, I go to the gym or do theatrical activities. After the break, you have to go back to the wing. There you can play table-football, ping-pong, various recreational activities, cards, tournaments with cards, or you can even cook. We have an electric hotplate, an electric oven, and another hotplate for toasting. Sometimes, up in Cassiopea, where the staff and the doctors went to great lengths to get us an extra hotplate, we can even make pizza. I managed to make pizza for everybody in the wing here, with the help of the guards who let me use the kitchen there in Cassiopea where I made pizza for everyone. In the evening they lock us up, give us our treatment, meals are served at noon and half past six in the evening. They give us the treatment at eight in the morning, at noon and in the evening. I only take it in the morning and in the evening. The purely psychiatric treatment only in the evening. I take ridiculously small doses, but this is relative. I'm not an ex-druggie or alcoholic. I take 5 mg of Zyprexa and 500 mg of Depakin, which is a lot for me. I'm a zombie in the morning, then after ten o' clock I get my act together and I want to do lots of things, most of which I can't do because there isn't the equipment here. There isn't a real rehab course and there's no structured organization in the FPH so that you can pursue a profession; if you're eligible, then you can do it outside the FPH when your term of imprisonment is over.

I Do Theater to Get ROTLs (Releases on Temporary License)

It was the doctor who advised me to do theater as it would accelerate the process for obtaining ROTLs. I got thirteen ROTLs by doing these theatrical activities, but now I'm on stand-by for tomorrow's show. I should be on. If the licenses arrive by tomorrow I'll be on, otherwise I can't leave the FPH. It depends on the magistrate because I'm a prisoner and inmate confined to this structure. In my case, the psychiatric rehabilitation technician makes the application to the magistrate. Then there are the psychiatric patients who've been acquitted, that's a difficult word, maybe we'll talk about that later. In their case it depends on the psychiatric institute with ministerial-juridical supervision and that means the police. These licenses are the responsibility of the ward doctor and the chief medical officer, and they are renewed automatically. For us 148s it's not like that; they have to check the reports on the previous licenses to see if everything went well and then get the psychiatrist's opinion, to check that the license did the patient some good, if it contributed to—let's say—a real or fictitious rehabilitative, psycho-physical and attitudinal state, or whether it didn't help at all. To recap, you can get these licenses, but they are benefits, they aren't rights. Just benefits.

This theatre business? No… I don't enjoy it. I go because I promised the lady that runs the theatre. They think doing theatre is useful, but I don't see it. In the meantime, I get licenses but this escamotage hasn't really been all that useful because the licenses aren't coming. My dream is to be an inmate with article 21, that gives you the benefit of working on the outside and coming back in the evening. You go out in the morning and come back in the evening at given times; you can even take a half hour to get a breath of air. There, that's what I'd really like. Since I've been here in Reggio Emilia I've had some benefits.

FPH, a Dumping Ground for Broken Humans

It's a structure where they collect… garbage, scum. There is human garbage, this is a dumping ground for human garbage. People who are not accepted because they are considered socially dangerous, or maybe because someone has decided that it's convenient that they are considered socially dangerous. In the past, usually the nobility (persons covered, protected, by nobility) were able to avoid Mental Hospitals. Between the end of the 1800s and the beginning of the 1900s there were places where they took people who were considered to be in one way or another, because they didn't conform to the canons of European, western or overseas, American civilizations. But these people protected by nobility didn't usually end up there, except for those cases where it was in someone's interests: they were labelled as schizophrenic so they could be locked up and their wealth taken away, so maybe we should refer to the central and peripheral nervous system through the phrenic nerve that stops functioning correctly and so causes people to behave a little despotically and say things in an overbearing way. But I don't want to teach you your job, of course!

If they were to send me outside, send me to Turin, I wouldn't be able to do a thing.

I'm not from Turin. I'm from Los Angeles, but I was born in New York City. I told you that at the beginning. If I get on to a sailing boat I remember how to navigate, even if I can't remember the names of all the parts of the boat.

My memory is confused…

Then there was Marco Cavallo; it was very emotional, very moving, but nothing changed inside the Structure, we still live with the same restrictions as before. But it was nice that someone came from the outside and brought us the blue horse, very, very nice. They did a lot in 1973 with the Trieste FPH, they broke down the walls and opened the doors of the FPH… however, there too… the mentally ill were thrown out into the street, there was no rehabilitation, just as there isn't any today. That's why I want to have article 21, so that I can have a rehabilitation course. I'm not an American citizen any longer, I'm Italian, I want to become a model Italian citizen, who has a conscience, who can work, a commitment to society as well as to a profession, as a voluntary worker. When I get a passport, I'll decide what to do. That's it. I've nothing more to add.

Mattia: The Mother and the Prostitutes

I Didn't Talk to Anyone

I used to be very ill, but that's in the past. Now I feel fine, I'm happy here, I want to continue with the positive rehabilitation course I'm on.

My malaise, distress brought me here from prison. I was very introverse, I wasn't like I am now. I didn't talk to anybody. The prisons I've been in? Aosta, Saluzzo, Cuneo, Porto Azzurro. I didn't talk to anyone in any of them, not to the inmates or the guards.

I've changed because I thought over what happened at Porto Azzurro. I realized I'd been in the wrong. One day I exploded and smashed up my cell.

I had those symptoms where you hear everything amplified. For some time, I thought that everyone had it in for me, they were talking about their own affairs, their own things…

Socially dangerous? I think that should apply to people who are dangerous, who behave badly, show signs of being disturbed, who can cause trouble, then they should be classified as socially dangerous.

I'm classified as socially dangerous, I hope someday they'll cancel it because I don't show signs of being disturbed any more, I'm not like I was then, then I was unbalanced… when I was in Porto Azzurro… not when I was in Montelupo, no, because at the beginning I was heavily sedated. The more medicine they gave me, the more violent I became.

When they stopped giving me medicine, I started to think things through, I realized that I'd been wrong and that I shouldn't have reacted like that.

I was really in a bad way when I was in Porto Azzurro, there was that episode of the cell. I'd never been in treatment before.

I wasn't well because I hated prostitutes. My mother was a prostitute and she treated me badly. She wanted me dead. She used to say, "When are you going to die?". Her father always compared me to my father and so I committed some murders. First, I killed a man, he was a *mafioso*, and afterwards I killed three prostitutes because they behaved like …

I killed the *mafioso* because he said to me, "If you don't do what I tell you to do, I'll have you killed". So I killed him. With a knife. I killed the prostitutes because they behaved like my mother. They blackmailed me, they swore at me, "If you don't come with us, we'll tell your wife you go with prostitutes". I see my mother in them, but not in all of them. Many of them were good people. I happened on three evil ones and I killed them. With a pistol.

The crimes I committed were hate crimes. I became mentally ill in prison, in Porto Azzurro in fact.

I've got a son but he doesn't write to me anymore, I think he doesn't want to have anything more to do with me.

My priest comes to see me. He's already come to visit twice since I've been here.

People Have Been a Greater Help to Me Than the Treatment

The transition from prison to the FPH helped me to think. At the beginning I was bad, they sedated me heavily in Montelupo. I wasn't myself and I was heavily sedated, then when they started to lighten the dose… even when I was full of medication I behaved myself, I talked to them, they helped me. The doctors and the lady doctor, they helped me. I started thinking things over and figured out where I'd been wrong.

People have been a greater help to me than medication. They stopped giving me the injections, they stopped the Serenase, they stopped a lot of the medication, before I was having injections, Serenase, Seroquel…

Now I just take 150 milligrams of Seroquel in the evening to help me sleep, I take some Valium and a little Risperdal and that's all. It's really very little. This is the place I like best. I've done theater here. And I do other sorts of activities too, I've never been to the newsletter, I think that's on Monday. What about the future? I haven't anyone on the outside. I'd like to stay here, unless something happens to make me change my mind… once my time is up, I don't know if they will send me away.

With early release I've still got two years and nine months to do. If I get a pardon, I'll just have a year and a bit still to do. After, there's the Care and Surveillance Facility but I don't know if I'll have to go there or whether they'll convert it to care in a Rehabilitation Community or some other structure.

I arrived here on August 10, 2011, that'll be three years this coming June and I like it here, because they welcomed me. They welcomed me like a relative, well, maybe that's a bit of an exaggeration, but that's what it felt like.

The psychiatrists, the nurses, the operators, really, they treat me and the others very well. Every week the doctor comes round to hear if there are any problems, to see if you need anything. It's fine here; the food? The food is good.

I've been in the FPH at Montelupo Fiorentino too, but it's different to here. It was OK there too, but the doctor didn't do the rounds every week like he does here, that's the only difference. The building there is old, a bit uglier, things don't function as well, there were more people to a room, and then you have someone who sees things in a certain way and others who see them differently. It was a bit like that. Here the wards are open until eight in the evening, there they were locked at six. There were more options for rehab: they had the newsletter, theater, things like that. I spent five or six years in Montelupo and three here. I've been in prison too and I got sick there, in Porto Azzurro on Elba. I arrived at Porto Azzurro in January 1999 and I got sick so they gave me article 148.[91]

I'm from the Val D'Aosta, I lived in small villages.

They were good in Porto Azzurro too, but I got sick and they put medication in my ear, then I stuck in a cotton bud and I heard everything amplified and I got sick. I was introverted, irascible, sullen. I heard voices in the corridor, really loud voices, and I thought there was something wrong with me but there wasn't. Then I recovered and the problem disappeared.

I came to the FPH with article 148 because I'd smashed up my cell, all because of that problem I had.

After that I haven't had any bad problems with my head.

I like it here in Reggio Emilia. It's a bit like a little family, I don't agree with the others about the structure but we discuss things, we socialize, the others complain a lot, about things they shouldn't be complaining about. I don't complain about things if there's no reason to.

The Structure is new, they treat you well, the food is good, you can eat well, I don't see anything to complain about.

---

[91] Article 48 of the Italian Penal Code states that if a person convicted of a crime develops a mental illness before the sentence restricting their personal freedom is executed, or during its execution, and the judge deems that the illness is such as to prevent the execution of the sentence, the sentence may be deferred or suspended and the convicted person sent to a Forensic psychiatric hospital, or to a specially designated nursing home.

I Attend Mass and Participate in the Group

The Care and Surveillance Facility, a residence for people who have committed crimes, people who are ill.

I realize that I wasn't well, they sent me to the FPH at Montelupo and then here to treat me, I get on very well with the psychiatrist, he takes good care of me, now they are working to get me a license, they got me a pardon, early release, monitored by the operators, I can't honestly complain about anything, I can't say anything against this place.

A typical day: I attend Mass, I go to the rosary meetings, to the deaconry, sometimes I go to the Ground Floor but I don't really like going there because there are some people who are a little … you can pay some money and buy whatever you want, honey, Coca Cola, brioches, it's very nice! In Montelupo there wasn't a bar, the Ground Floor; there you just had time in the yard, but life was OK there too, they weren't unkind at all.

I get on very well with don Daniele. He's very good, understanding and always accessible. Participating in the group helps me a lot.

Mario: "Schizoaffectivity" and Feelings

My Beloved Dogs

They were talking on the news about people who want to change their name because of difficulties like psychological plots…that film *Tutta colpa di Freud* (All Freud's fault).

In this photo here behind, you can get a glimpse of the school of art and culture I went to, it's a CPF (a Center for Professional Training). I took my father's mother's surname. And for reasons looking for their origins, I ended up taking refuge here, in the FPH of Reggio Emilia. My father's mother was my last grandmother to die. I took my first steps in psychiatry after meeting this Danish woman. I was at Lake Garda. That's how my father met my mother, who is from Puglia. During the war my father was a Swiss partisan and worked as a simultaneous translator. Sometimes, even if the words seem intertwined or don't make sense, there are alternative depths of recognition, sometimes nothing else is understood. As the poorest boy I had my moments of toxicity and I opened the doors of perception and shared it with my dogs. [Shows the photos]. This is my father; he was a runner, a great sportsman. Don't even mention Cindy Crawford who is always a sight for sore eyes.

This is me in the Rehab center, I was a bit overweight. This is Shakira, she was called that at the beginning when the song *Whenever, wherever* came out. In 2003.

Now eleven-twelve years ago, *Shakira the she-wolf wants a son* has come out.

There are coincidences that when you understand them… you call on the origins where you have strengthened yourself, you get strength from the origins where you have cultivated them. The tones of multimedia ways, sometimes you are in a time of reasons and intersections in a direct line with the acknowledgement of a cathodic tube…

Let's take a step back… regarding the screen. Every day I search for karma for my interior peace, which lies in my dogs, Sunday, Harlock, Shakira.

I arrived here in 2007, from June 2007 to June 2008. Resisting arrest. Acquitted for insanity. Acquitted.

I had an accident in 2005, a car cut across me, didn't give way, I crashed: my femur was fractured, I have a femoral reduction, without this nail they'd have to do another operation, the left leg is already 3 to 4 centimeters short. Later I found out from the other party's forensic expert that I'd broken my jaw and the bridge of my nose. After the operation I took Shakira for a walk and she mated with a setter crossed with a Neapolitan Mastiff, that's why Sunday and Harlock are so different, Yin and Yang they were, Harlock is all black with white paws. These here in the photo … Now that's something I've never been able to accept… one of the puppies didn't survive birth and she, my mother, got rid of it. I guess it was born dead.

After my accident Sunday was born, Sunday that sounds a bit like "some day".

Harlock is blind in one eye, the Capitan Harlock of the comic strips.

I had four other operations in March 2005, after the accident.

I spent Easter, Christmas, my birthday, Saint Valentine's in the meantime up to 2007 when there was a fork in the ways of everything took on another direction, another meaning. There, my story started with her …

I Met Her, "Schizoaffectivity"

My psychiatric experience started after I met her. The "*Schizoaffectivity*". I spent six months locked up in a psychiatric ward.

In the morning I went to prune the vines, I'd saved a bit of money to go and see her, in Holdborg. I was thinking about going to visit her there. It was an objective, a goal I'd set myself, to go see her... I'd even written some poetry, I'd met a girl in one of the four or five Rehab Centers I've been in, before I was in a Community because I was under articles 206–208 as socially dangerous. I met Astrid, she was born on 10/10/1984. My brother was born on 5/5/1984. Kind of odd, isn't it?

I don't have the chance to do anything creative... with the money I should get as compensation. I've got a lawyer, but I don't really understand the situation about the inheritance...I'd meant to use, see this is a farm ... I tell you what a friend of mine said, he's an art director who became a policeman in Verona and that one day when I was in the FPH the inspector called to say that my mother had been taken to a psychiatric ward because she'd had a nervous breakdown. This art director friend took care of everything, my mother had five dogs and my brother and this friend said, "I'll put them in a farm". After I got out of the Rehab I went to see them...

It's not easy, bringing everything up. It was great to see the dogs. In fact it was emotional. Maybe I can do something for the farm with the compensation money... Sometimes you can communicate a word with your eyes and soul without having to speak it.

I'd like to leave here ... and find a way to take the room I have ...

My little project is to take up a gym, one of those bench presses with everything, just for a start, the most difficult part is to stop drinking, a depurative period... like Karaoke evenings, I started from scratch, went out clubbing... maybe I want to keep it inside me.

This is Bossi. When I was in high school, he came to see the work we did, sculpting stone... now as a last step to get out of here I've asked my lawyer to come, to get a report with the medical examiner as well as finding my autonomy... seeing as how it seems I'm not in full possession of my faculties and can't vote... sorry, I'd set the alarm...

4

The Forensic Psychiatric Hospital of Barcellona Pozzo Di Gotto

The Forensic Psychiatric Hospital of Barcellona Pozzo di Gotto

The Forensic Psychiatric Hospital of Barcellona Pozzo di Gotto in the province of Messina on the island of Sicily was the last FPH to be closed. At the beginning of April 2017, three years after the decision to close these structures and transform them into REMS, and two months from the official announcement that all the inmates had been successfully reassigned, there were still four patients in residence in Barcellona Pozzo di Gotto. They were the last of a group of fifteen for whom the authorities were having difficulty in finding new destinations. Franco Corleone, who had been the sole Commissioner for the Government for the winding up of the FPHs since February 2016, announced, "Now it is only a question of a few days. The measures already approved by the Department of Prison Administration should be activated by Monday: two of the inmates will go to the REMS in Barete, Abruzzo, one will be put on parole in Sicily or will go to a REMS here, and one will be transferred to a structure in Modena, where he has his residence." Notwithstanding this, it wasn't until May 11, 2017 that the last inmate of Barcellona Pozzo di Gotto was

J. Santambrogio, *Stories from Italian Forensic Psychiatric Hospitals*,
https://doi.org/10.1007/978-3-031-61129-2_4

finally accepted by a therapeutic community in Modica, Sicily. On his report, Corleone wrote, "Today will go down in history as the day on which the era of internment in these totalitarian institutions is finally closed and the grim names of Aversa, Montelupo, Reggio Emilia, Secondigliano are consigned to the memory of a past that must never be allowed to return. Castiglione delle Stiviere, too, must adhere to this reform that has decreed the closure of the FPHs and the abandoning of the concept of mental asylums. Italy can be proud of being in the forefront of this field in Europe and in the world; after the closure of the Civil Mental Asylums in compliance with Law 180, we are now facing the most difficult task of all, the cancellation of the horror of the Criminal Mental Asylums."[1]

Barcellona Pozzo di Gotto was the fifth FPH to come into existence, after Aversa (1876), Montelupo Fiorentino (1886), Reggio Emilia (1892), Napoli (1923). It was inaugurated on May 6, 1925; among those present was Alfredo Rocco, the Minister of Justice of the time who was later to revise and append his signature to the Penal Code and the Penal Procedure Code (1930), subsequently known as the *Codice Rocco* or Rocco Code. The idea of constructing an FPH in Barcellona Pozzo di Gotto originated in 1904 during Giovanni Giolitti's second government and the foundation stone was laid in May 1908. Work on the building was interrupted by the deadly earthquake that devastated Messina and Reggio Calabria in December 1908, so it was not completed until 1919. It was declared habitable a few years later.

The history of the construction and first years of activity of the FPH has been written in painstaking detail by Vittorio Madia, nominated director of the institution on March 28, 1929, in a report for the *Rivista di Diritto Penitenziario*.[2] Madia was the Chief Psychiatrist of the Naples Mental Asylum, "where he stood out for his exceptional professional capacity". He was assigned to direct, organize and restructure Barcellona Pozzo di Gotto after two brief and disastrous attempts by other directors.

[1] Corleone, F. (2017). Chiusi gli OPG, ora mai più Manicomi. *Rubrica di Fuoriluogo, Il Manifesto*.

[2] Madia, V. (1932). Il Manicomio Giudiziario di Barcellona Pozzo di Gotto. *Rivista di Diritto Penitenziario: Studi teorici e pratici*. Anno III, n. 4 Luglio-Agosto. pp. 1019–1316. http://digitale.bnc.roma.sbn.it/tecadigitale/visore/#/main/viewer?idMetadato=17236381&type=bncr.

Madia took over on April 4, 1929, and rapidly transformed the institution, introducing an efficient work methodology and innovative ways of treating the patients. In his 25 years as director, Madia elevated Barcellona Pozzo di Gotto to the level of the European and American institutions, receiving the "Best in Italy" award. It became a model institution, to the extent that in 1954 the Minister of Justice called Madia to Rome and entrusted him with the task of organizing the new FPH wing of the prison of Rebibbia. He left Sicily on October 31 for Rome, but this new mission was not to be, he died on November 27, 1954. Madia firmly believed that liberty and work were the fundamental ingredients for rehabilitation, and so organized a vast range of activities, from carpentry to the cultivation of lemons and oranges, from the creation of an atelier for tailoring and a bookbinding laboratory to workshops, ironworking, cobbling. He also opened a library, and, for the first time in Italy, set up a primary school classroom in an FPH equipped with desks, blackboard, maps, and a radio. In 1932, twenty-four inmates sat their exams in the presence of a commission chaired by the Didactic Director of the State primary schools and obtained their certification. Every year there were new, stimulating activities for the inmates. In 1951 Professor Benigno Tullio, the Director of the only Institute of Criminal Anthropology in Italy, visited Barcellona Pozzo di Gotto and recorded his impressions with the following statement, "I am extraordinarily pleased to have visited an FPH which is a model of technical organization. But more than this, my sincerest appreciation and highest praise go to our worthy colleague Madia, who with his lively intellect, sense of care and perfect scientific knowledge has created this model FPH which brings honor to Italy and the science of criminology".

A wing for mentally handicapped inmates and a *Casa di Cura e Custodia* for inmates with special needs were added in 1945 and 1969 respectively. During this period the Institution was named after its illustrious director, Vittorio Madia.

In the years that followed, Barcellona Pozzo di Gotto fell on bad times and was associated with cases of degradation. Indeed, in 2010 Ignazio Marino, the President of a Parliamentary Commission investigating the efficiency and efficacy of the National Health Service, visited the FPH and reported finding "a completely naked man bound with strips of cloth to an iron bed with a rusty hole in the center for the release of urine and feces."

The last detailed social-health report on the FPH of Barcellona Pozzo di Gotto was drawn up by the *Associazione Antigone*[3] and dates back to March 30, 2015, when the FPH was under the management of Dr. Nunziante Rosania. At that time, the FPH was still functioning and housed 156 inmates, cared for by 4 doctors, 10 psychiatrists and 70 nurses. The report states, "At the time of our visit, many of the inmates have voluntarily stated that they do not want to be transferred to other structures, this either because they have already been in other rehabilitation centers and were not happy there, or simply because they don't want to lose the relationships they have forged here with the health workers and prison staff, and start all over again in a different environment". It continues, "A form of dynamic surveillance has been in force in the FPH for a number of years. The inmates can move freely within the ward from 0.800 to 22.30 and can go out frequently into the courtyard next to their ward (the schedule is flexible, each ward has its own timetable). The single and multiple occupancy cells are almost always left open, except in the case of single cells when the inmate has been isolated temporarily (ward 3) or for health reasons. During our visit only a few doors were shut, but because the inmates themselves wanted them so. There are telecameras in almost all the wards and the management made a point of explaining that under no circumstances can a prison guard remain alone with an inmate, at least one health worker must always be present. During our visit the relations between the prison guards and the inmates appeared relaxed and serene, certainly helped by the fact that the inmates can move about freely in the wards, so sharing space with the guards.

The prison guards themselves consider that working with open cells is a great advantage as it defuses tensions and internal conflicts. Many, who have worked in the FPH for many years, remarked on the substantial difference between this structure and traditional prisons, judging the

[3] Associazione Antigone is an association founded in 1991, whose social purpose is the protection of the rights of prisoners and the raising of awareness of issues related to prisons and incarceration.

working conditions here to be much better. The health workers too are all in all satisfied with this system of freedom in the wards, and it appears that their relationship with most of the inmates is very tranquil."[4]

Diary of the Visits

February 17: Day 1. As already explained in the Introduction, I visited Barcellona Pozzo di Gotto in February 2013, staying in Padre Pippo's halfway house for seven days, rubbing shoulders with inmates on probation, to consult with them on how best to structure my project.

Two Sicilian friends gave me a lift to the halfway house and left me outside the massive front doors holding an offering of marzipan cakes. The doors opened and I was drawn inside by a group of burly, well-built men who then moved aside to reveal Padre Pippo, frail in body but great at heart.

Dinner was at 19.30; everyone sat quietly around a long table and Padre Pippo, at the head of the table, said grace. I had been expecting a raucous atmosphere, but the reality was quite different, it was almost like being in a monastery. There was also the mother of one of the inmates who had come to visit her son and was staying in the halfway house. "He was never right, not even at home, "she explained. "He would say he was in touch with the Son of God and that he wanted to go to Jerusalem to be with his brothers. Then one day he took one of our kitchen knives and went over to his father who was sitting on the sofa watching television and pointed it under his chin. It was a miracle my husband didn't die. That's why my son ended up here in Barcellona". After dinner I had my first conversations with the inmates, settled comfortably on couches in the living room, and took notes. "It all depends on the cell you end up in. I was in a cell with a guy who had really bad schizophrenia, he swallowed light bulbs and metal locks so they would send him to the Infirmary. I had a PR agency, I organized events, then… two punches, a fight and

[4] Ospedale Psichiatrico Giudiziario Barcellona Pozzo di Gotto "Vittorio Madia". Report of the Associazione Antigone on March 30, 2015. https://www.antigone.it/upload2/uploads/docs/OPGVisite.pdf.

they sent me to the Ucciardone for a week. After, they sent me to the FPH, I didn't even know such a thing existed. It's a prison, but they give you pills. Then there is this system of extensions; we are fighting the judiciary, Jacopo!". Another inmate had a different point of view, "Life in the FPH is grim. It's not a hospital, it's a prison, it's not a place where you can get better, it's a place where you get worse because it's a closed environment and you are shut in with sick people. Then you don't get the correct therapy, how can a psychiatrist give you the right medicine after exchanging just a few words with you? These are hellholes". Another inmate asked if he could have a word. He's spent twenty-three years in a high security prison and was in his fourth in the FPH, where he worked as a cook and gardener. He was on a five-day permit with Padre Pippo.

February 18: Day 2. Padre Pippo, during a long interview that took place in his studio, gave me a detailed overview of the complex story of the Barcellona FPH and the timeline of its closure. He then accompanied me to the FPH and, pointing to the walls, remarked, "There used to be guards all long these walls". We met a friend of the priest's, a psychiatrist, but I was soon called away to a meeting with Dr. Rosania, who gave me a cordial welcome and mentioned that some of the inmates would be lunching with him later. "They're having lunch with you at home?", I asked. "Yes," came the answer, "my wife is involved in some activities with them. Later I'll stop by the halfway house to organize the program for the week".

February 19: Day 3. Another session with Padre Pippo in the morning, this time on the origins and the history of the halfway house. He then called the Director to organize a tour of the FPH for me, in the company of a psychiatrist. Accessing the FPH was no easy matter as I didn't have a written authorization, but after a number of phone calls I was allowed inside. The guard on the desk was particularly kind as she saw from my identity card that we were both born in Carate Brianza, well over a thousand kilometers away. Once inside the walls, I was impressed by the layout of the garden and the avenues of orange trees; the psychiatrist pointed out some murals painted by the inmates, his favorite was the last of the line, a human figure with the wording, "An empty head looking for…".

We went up the stairs to the Fifth Ward. A bit squalid, at first glance. A reinforced door, a guard standing at attention and a group of inmates moving around in the corridor. I will never forget those faces. Maybe Lombroso had something, with his theory of anthropological criminology. We visited the infirmary where the chief nurse and a health worker were carefully and seraphically selecting and folding what looked like scraps of material. They were doing this because some of the inmates had nothing to wear. They seemed worn down by years and years of work in this place, and, at least at a first glance, they looked as if they really cared. The visits started with N. (a murderer). N. spoke easily, fluently, very wrapped up in a soliloquy expressing his anger at the forthcoming transfer to another ward. We moved on to talk to A., a man with a friendly face and scars on the nape of his neck from banging against the walls in protest, and an another on his neck, an old wound from self-harming with a broken bottle. He also had marks of recent cuts on his arms; not long before our visit he had smashed up the bathroom because a psychiatrist had modified the therapy prescribed by *his* doctor. After this, he said, "I was locked into the solitary confinement cell for twenty-four hours, naked, with only a bed without sheets or blankets". He had been in the FPH for eleven years for sexually assaulting his sister-in-law. "I've made it up with my brother," he said, "but not with my sister-in law". He has all the symptoms of a severe mental disability. When he looks at you there is cunning in his glance, but at the same time there is something perverse, sick. When we left, he called out, "Ciao, Jacopo!".

The last visit is to V., who is wearing an elegant jacket and has a pleasant face and a frank, open expression. "This is man's talk, doctor, I can't say it in front of you". The psychiatrist moved away, and V. confided that when he urinates he has a burning sensation and passes blood. I examined his medical records and saw there had been a number of recent consultations, so I reassured him that he was being appropriately cared for. V. stood up and tried to hug the health worker, who stiffened up somewhat. His medical records indicated that he "suffers from epilepsy, is intellectually challenged, graft-psychosis" and he was being treated with Luminal (an anti-epileptic), Tegretol and Haldol depot, to counteract his elevated impulsivity. V. was in the FPH for sexual violence.

Cigarettes, for the inmates, are a question of life and death. You can have committed a crime of sexual violence like A., be confined in the FPH and continue to be (or pretend to be) mentally disturbed because you don't get the cigarettes you are entitled to. So it was essential that the health workers kept a detailed record of how the cigarettes were distributed.

February 20: Day 4. Today should have been the day that the FPH closed its doors forever, but it didn't. Quite the contrary, a theatrical representation had been organized for the inmates.

I spoke to Carmela, one of the voluntary workers, about the therapeutical potential of theatrical activities for psychiatric patients. Carmela met Padre Pippo when he was the priest for Santa Lucia del Mela and she was a voluntary worker in an adoption center for minors. She admitted that "FPHs as such should no longer exist. There is a problem regarding the people who work there, because they are not office workers, they deal with human beings who have a right to be treated as such. They have their dignity. Padre Pippo has fought incessantly for the closure of these places, which he considers to be inhuman, and finally he has succeeded."

In the FPH we met a psychiatrist with the opposite view regarding the closure. He claimed he had cured some of the inmates and their relatives had been truly grateful. He believed in the FPH and was opposed to shutting them down. "Where will they send these people who have committed serious crimes now?". We went on to visit an inmate suffering from schizophrenia. The psychiatrist immediately adjusted to the patient, entering into harmony with him but laughing at him at the same time. I learned later that he had a heavy hand when prescribing medication.

We watched the play. One of the actors was a nineteen-year-old foreigner who had killed a senator but was completely oblivious to the crime he had committed. There were many inmates in the audience. As the curtain went down, Padre Pippo spoke a few words, "We've managed it, finally. The FPH is to be closed." On the way out I met a prison guard who was contrary to the closure. He was very agitated and was intent on telling me his point of view. "Where will they put the murderers and all the people who commit serious offences? This place performs a function. Why do they say that it doesn't work if 60% of the inmates can be released? How will these new structures deal with really dangerous inmates?". I watched a prison guard supervising the return to the wards: rough with the inmates to exert his authority, pleasant to the doctor and to me.

February 21: Day 5. I had breakfast in the coffee shop with G. He asked me, "Do you eat at McDonald's or Burger King? Maybe too often? We don't have them here". We chatted about food and the problems related to food as G. was quite evidently overweight.

Today I had a meeting with Dr. Rosania, and we commented on the play performed yesterday. The theater has great cathartic potential and promotes reflection on the condition of the inmates, life in a cell, cohabitation and cigarettes. The ignorance of both inmates and doctors was represented with irony.

I had been impressed by the speech the Director had made from the stage at the beginning of the event. He had stated that the FPH as such is no longer in line with the times, "Barcellona Pozzo di Gotto is, to all extents and purposes, a prison. It is impossible to practice a good standard of psychiatry in these conditions. Practicing psychiatry implies reconstructing the person's social fabric, administering the appropriate therapy, reconstructing a normal habitat. Prisons, created as a safeguard for society, are synonymous with marginality, exclusion. Prisons and psychiatry are incompatible. Why do these places still exist? They are social rubbish dumps. Finally, our politicians have accepted this. Measures have been taken, albeit not enough. Our objective is to accommodate these people and support them in a decent environment. Our prison guards have never been trained to deal with psychiatric problems and have come into contact with some very difficult situations. They deserve respect and appreciation for this. The FPH will now be converted into a prison, as this territory needs a seat of legality".

February 22: Day 6. Today was interesting also from the clinical point of view.

9:30. I was on the point of going into Padre Pippo's office when one of the guests, a certain K., started shouting at Carmela and telling her to "Shut up!". He became more and more aggressive, yelling insults at both Padre Pippo and Carmela. He has been waiting for a permit for four months and his social assistant had promised to bring him news of it the day before. Carmela tried to calm him down, but K. grabbed a chair, hurled it against a cupboard, then against the photocopier and made to attack Carmela. I stepped between them, told him, "We are friends", and managed to convince him to leave the room with me. Outside, sitting on a bench, K. was in tears. He was still very agitated, and said he wanted to smash something, maybe the computer, destroy it. He can't stand the waiting, and the continuous delays. He was a soldier, possibly a leader, and a political refugee. His story is long, complicated and disturbing. He was certainly suffering from depression, anxiety, probably due to traumatic experiences and emotive fragility. He swings from tears to slightly idiotic laughter and has outbursts of violent rage.

Finally, the social assistant arrives, called by Padre Pippo. She is very concerned as she is convinced the permit hasn't arrived. K. loses his temper again and calls her *macaca e zigzaga*, which means a person who doesn't keep their promises. We all go to the police station, where K. loses his temper again, but fortunately there is another social assistant there who has a better relationship with him (maybe a transfert, maybe he sees his dead sister in her). After a long wait, the permit is finally produced and we all return to the halfway house. I check K.'s medication: he is taking Depakin (500 mg ½ + ½), Solian (400 mg × 2), Tavor (2.5 mg × 2), Diazepam (30 drops × 3). Maybe not enough for a soldier suffering from war trauma. Maybe a selective serotonin reuptake inhibitor would help? His psychiatrist says to add another Solian at midday.

Later, in the FPH I was present at a meeting between the Director and the father and sister of S., who had killed his mother ten years previously, stabbing her 97 times. Paranoid schizophrenia, with the conviction that other people could read his mind, exacerbated by LSD and cannaboids taken in high school. He had lived in symbiosis with his mother and father, expanded ego and significant obsessivity.

February 23: Day 7. Ward 8, first floor. Padre Pippo is interviewing the candidates for the trip outside the FPH, planned for the following Wednesday. There are inmates who have longed for the opportunity to go on this trip and have the requisites, others who have longed to go but don't have the requisites and are angry and frustrated, others who have the requisites but don't want to go. In fact, there are inmates who have been in the FPH for years but have never set a foot outside because they are happy where they are, and are convinced that "just a little longer and I'll be leaving anyway".

Dr. Aldo Madia invited me to accompany him on his rounds to visit some inmates, taking great pains to show me the various therapies. He worked in pharmacology in Pisa for several months and is very well prepared.

We saw D. who tried to negotiate his medication and variations to his therapy. He is guilty of extortion, illegal possession of firearms. He got on the wrong side of someone in his village and he is back here again.

M. attends an IT course every morning. He likes to keep his hand in. He has a kind face; the nurses say he sleeps all the time.

D.N., an unlicensed parking attendant from Catania, is in the FPH because while conducting his parking business he stole a car in (unauthorized) exchange for the scooter someone stole from him. Unfortunately for him he got caught. He is a delightful character. He worked as a plumber in the morning and in the afternoon parked cars (again without the necessary authorization). He refuses to take his midday medication. Dr. Madia gave him Serenase in drops.

F., who has eyes as blue as the sea around Sicily, is severely retarded mentally. He was remanded to the FPH for a grievous sexual attack on a minor.

P. is a gentle soul from the city of Lecce. He has been in Barcellona for two years on a provisional security measure, waiting to go on trial for threatening his father and beating him up. Dr. Madia explained that "there are crimes for which the offenders would normally get a two-year security measure, but as they don't have enough money to pay a lawyer, and the lawyer assigned by the court is maybe slow in filing the papers, they can be detained up to five years on provisional security measures. What is really absurd is that, if you have a good lawyer, you could be acquitted as being unfit to plead and not even be declared to be a danger to society. You go scot-free without doing a day in FPH or other forms of detention".

This period in Barcellona Pozzo di Gotto with Padre Pippo, Aldo Madia and the inmates of the FPH laid the foundation for the project and prepared me, professionally and psychologically, for the meetings and interviews of the following year.

Martino: Confabulation and The Korsakoff Syndrome

We Were All There Together with Vallanzasca[5]

We'll talk about prison because I've done lots of that, as well as thirteen years of FPH. And some time in rehab centers. Life inside, in prison, well, there's less confusion than there is here in the FPH. What I mean is, there is less intimacy with the other inmates. There is less of that in prison because the inmates tend to mind their p's and q's because there's a law that cites this article, I think it was the Vassalli law, no, wait, it was the Gozzini, the Gozzini law.[6] Before the Martelli. An expert? Me? No, I read the papers and then I was inside. Prisoners tend to mind their step.

In 1971 we were all inside, like that famous guy, you know, Renato Vallanzasca. In those years we were all together in one institution or another. We got together and demonstrated against the Martelli law[7] because it didn't allow for a yearly reduction of your sentence, not like the Gozzini law; well, our protests got the Martelli law overturned and we all did our bit to get our sentences extended for having participated in all those protests over the years.

In '73, in the 1980s, in 2006 they handed out amnesties, and they gave out pardons but I didn't get one because I was a habitual offender.

The difference, I'm going back to your question, between the FPH and prison is that there is more confusion in the FPH in the sense that you are at the mercy of the pathologies of your companions, you have to live at 80 cm one from another. In those days we were 8, 10, 11 to a cell. I'm talking about the Aversa FPH. I was there under observation, I came from prison because I was in Favignana where I was doing manual work. Well, see, in their opinion I had a bit of *mental illness. Caused by alcohol.*

---

[5] Renato Vallanzasca was a notorious Italian mobster who was a powerful figure in the Milanese underworld during the 1970s.

[6] The Gozzini law aimed at giving more importance to rehabilitation rather than punishment in prison.

[7] The protests to which Martino is referring were probably those of 2004 and 2008 against the chronic overcrowding in the prisons and modifications to the benefits/reductions of the sentence established by the Gozzini law.

I drank a bit in prison. Yep. I drank, half a liter of alcohol, wine or beer. All legal and above board, just that I overdid it. It's not the quarter of alcohol that you drink. It's that out of ignorance you try to see if you can get drunk. Ignorance leads to these sorts of things. Was I bored? Were we bored? No, don't think so. It's just you get yourself all revved up and challenge the alcohol to change you. But it takes years to figure out that it changes you. In fact, it does, alcohol does: easy writing under the influence. When I read and I wasn't high anymore I'd rip up the letters and didn't send them. They were all about "bring me this", "do that for me". Alcohol is a damned nuisance that you've got to get in hand.

I lost my mind to alcohol.

Talking to the guards, "You with the keys, you who can, open number 5 for me, number ten, will you?". "And what am I supposed to open, it isn't time!". Therefore, there was the crunch between *going out* and *not going out*. And so, protests.

I haven't finished with the difference between FPH and prison. In prison you put on an act so you get to go to the FPH to get acquitted. You pretend to be mad and that thirty years are too many. I've met people who've done this. I didn't because I just had 5 years and 6 months. Contempt, simulated offence, possession of a dangerous weapon, forcing a roadblock, that was on June 8, 1971, the second offence because I'd been had up in 1968 for stealing cattle.

I'm a Sicilian. No, I wasn't a breeder. My friends were out of work, I had a job, they asked me to come along on these robberies, they weren't violent robberies, they didn't cause any harm, we just took three, four lambs and then sold them to the shepherd. The shepherd knew us and ratted on us. We were arrested one after the other in Caltagirone in '67, '68. I was a minor, it was my first time inside, I got seven-eight months, I got isolation, I met lots of folk that gave you good stuff…

Anyway, to finish this about prisoners who make things up to get sent to the FPH. I never did this because I didn't need to, I didn't have thirty years to do. I was OK with staying in prison. I'd finish my three years and that would be that. But then we all did our bit—although it was wrong—to overturn the Martelli law with the Gozzini law, with guerilla tactics, throwing mattresses into the wards, refusing to go into the rooms. All that extended my sentence to almost forty years. I came out of that really badly.

The difference with the FPH, let's get this over with because we have to finish it. Simulated offence. The prisoner makes up stuff, and often the psychiatrist believes him. Why? Because he [the prisoner] goes the whole hog and simulates suicide, like he sticks a fork into his neck to make a mark that looks as if he was hanging himself. And then he shows off. He wants to have his thirty years in prison commuted into ten in the FPH. But that's a mistake because there are extensions to make sure you don't get out after ten years. They extend your sentence like they did to me, fourteen extensions I got.

On the 13th of this month, in Messina, they reviewed my situation. The lawyer told me that there aren't any Communities or rehab centers the judge can send me to, so when he finds a Community he'll send me there because I've never escaped from a Community, even though they wrote that I'm a person that apparently—this is written in black and white and recorded by the judge—is fine but actually has a dual personality. This is damaging. It's a wrong diagnosis. Because having a dual personality means that you aren't you. Therefore, you have delinquent intentions. With this dual personality, one is OK, the other, well, the other makes you commit … I don't know, robberies, for example. I'm not happy here in the FPH. I don't have psychiatric pathologies to compare with paranoids, schizophrenics, maniacs. I understand that because I read, listen, I get four news bulletins a day.

I've grown up in these unhealthy places, I take cardio aspirin, now I'm taking pills for my cholesterol, one for diabetes, one for my blood pressure. I'm sixty-five years old and I'm waiting for somewhere, a halfway house or a place where you aren't stuck behind a gate like you are here. You're not free here. I haven't got a family, I lost everything because the years were long and many. I'm sixty-five years old. I'm a survivor of these places. I know everything and everyone.

I Met Buscetta Too

They decided I wasn't a danger to society anymore but then they changed their mind after a year because I left my town. I was under house-arrest, I wasn't allowed to go out. One of my brothers committed suicide. His wife, my sister-in-law, she died and he committed suicide, hanging himself in the orchard. But that doesn't justify me leaving my town to go to the next one. Before that I'd committed other violations, so the judge threw me into prison: "A serious risk to society". There had been complaints about me, they said I played around a lot, molesting boys and girls and older women. It's true I'd stop the kids, they were playing on a football pitch, I knew their father, he was a marshal. That boy with all the other boys became my friends and when they saw me they'd call, "Uncle! Uncle!" and I said to them, "Off you go now, because the police don't want [me playing with you]".

For the police these reports were like setting off a time bomb to put me inside because a woman had been molested. It's true. I was put in therapeutic communities in Parma, then Turin Vallette, Genoa Marassi. I've been moving around since '71, that's forty years. I was put in the FPH when I finished my sentence in prison. Two years and eight months plus six for having a knife in prison. They didn't give me any time off. After that they sent me to Castelfranco Emilia as an inmate in a supervised working colony there. The psychiatrist got me a year in the *Rehab center* and sent me to the FPH. He had me taken away from the working colony because it was an agricultural community and it's easy to walk away from that but they sent me to Asinara in Sardinia. The sea is immense there.

Aversa in 1976. I was there under observation so I sawed one of the bars to escape. Ten months, I protested, "I'm not ill, I want to go back to prison". What happened after I sawed through the bar? They sent me back to Favignana, Favignana sent me off like a parcel in the post and I ended up in San Gimignano, a small room, you couldn't smash the glass in the windows, there was no oxygen, it was suffocating. There was one of the NAR,[8] a fascist, a certain Enrico. "What's your name?", he asked and threw me some cigarettes, coffee and a rolled-up magazine. I've met some really good people; I've met all sorts. I even met Buscetta in Palermo, the *mafioso* who is in the history books. He died, in Brazil, I think. He said to me, "Let's keep our noses clean". HE said that, to ME!

[8] The Nuclei Armati Rivoluzionari (Armed Revolutionary Nuclei), abbreviated NAR, was an Italian neo-fascist militant terrorist organization active during the so-called Years of Lead from 1977 to November 1981.

In April 1999 I ended up here in the FPH in Barcellona, but before that I did six years in Montelupo. Then I came here.

I Want to Get Out and Put All This Behind Me

You want to know if I'd find it difficult to live in the outside world? No, because there's work I can do. I'm a farmhand, but there's the term "independent farmer" or "agricultural laborer". I've got a certificate for metal working, demolition man. And shoemaker, I was a shoemaker in Volterra. Then I was an orderly in various prisons. I can survive in the outside world, no sweat. Last year they let me out to live in a halfway house near Parma. I got on well. I got back the driving license I'd lost, now they've taken it away because the insurance was faked. If they said to me, "Go and find a way of making your living outside of here", I'd go back to my town and I'd find somewhere to live and a job. Here it's difficult. I've been in a Rehab since the beginning of April. I've got a review on the 13th. My lawyer hasn't found any project or Rehab, when he does the judge will send me there. But the Social Services don't do anything right away, they'll let the extension expire. I'm working on it, I've been writing to the mayor of my town. Now all I want to do is to put the past behind me, because it's an experience of life and I need it like that. But I tell myself it wasn't a negative experience because I could have committed much more serious crimes than I did, as I was ignorant, not having had the benefit of culture from school. I haven't got a diploma, but I've learned plenty from life, but I'm not aggressive, I'm not a troublemaker, I listen a lot and I want others to listen to me if possible, otherwise we're not going to get on. I've an easy life, I haven't had a difficult life. If I get out, I don't want any help from the Social Services, I don't want them to find a project for me, because I'll find one for myself. And nothing else because otherwise I'll still be here when I'm seventy-five.

There is a difference between being a patient in the FPH and an inmate in prison. It's true that people with mental illnesses never get better, but I'm fine, why should I get ill? I've gotten over other people's pathologies by being a psychiatrist for them. I've got a certain background. Like now, I'm together with youngsters with schizophrenic and deliriant pathologies. It's not a dialogue between inmates, "Don't worry, I've got a pal who has a lot of land and we'll go and work there". This kind of conversation just doesn't exist in the FPH. Here there's the hate and the abandonment that there used to be in the mental asylums, because that is what these places are.

I experienced the Law 180 in Aversa, I went through that. I saw young guys with loss of memory: some prayed, some were tied up, some tied themselves under the bed. Me, no. They sent me there under observation for six months without any anti-psychotics. Under observation for six months. Me and five others, we weren't mad. All because a friend of mine made the mistake of pissing on a guard while he was sleeping.

Now I just want to get out of here and forget, to get back into the real world as soon as possible, find myself a family and forget all this. That's it. I've nothing else to say.

Reflections on Martino's Interview

What struck me about Martino was his smile, and the ironical look in his eyes that seemed to reflect on what his life had become. Forty years spent between prisons and FPH; his first experience of prison in a town in south-west Sicily when he was in his twenties, for having stolen some livestock.

His humble origins and lack of schooling were undoubtedly factors contributing to the *mistakes* he made along the way: driving without a license, theft, self-harming, attacks on minors, an attack on a woman. Martino listed these mistakes with little awareness of their significance. His story was confused, tangential, circumstantial, the associative connections weak.

"Life inside, in prison, well, there's less confusion than there is here in the FPH. What I mean is, there is less intimacy with the other inmates. There is less of that in prison because the inmates tend to mind their conduct because there's a law that cites this article, I think it was the Vassalli law, no, wait, it was the Gozzini, the Gozzini law. Before the Martelli. An expert? Me? No, I read the papers and then I was inside. Prisoners tend to mind their conduct." When asked about the difference between prison and FPH, Martino didn't start with an analysis of his personal experience, which he could well have done given that he has spent years in both types of institution, on the contrary he brought up his memories, fairly precise memories, regarding the legislative measures that regulate life in prison. In fact, the Gozzini law (Law n. 663 of October 10, 1986) aimed at enhancing the rehabilitative as opposed to the punitive aspects of detention and established a series of conditions for the authorization of permits and periods of probation, and so could well have encouraged Martino and his fellow prisoners to behave appropriately to obtain a reduction of their sentences for good conduct. Martino was particularly interested in this law because he was emotively involved in the fight for prisoners' rights. He went on to comment on his experiences, "In 1971 we were all inside, like that famous guy, you know, Renato Vallanzasca. In those years we were all together in one institution or another. We got together and demonstrated against the Martelli law because it didn't allow for a yearly reduction of the sentence, not like the Gozzini law; well, our protests got the Martelli law overturned and we all did our bit to get our sentences extended for having participated in all those protests over the years" but then the story becomes more and more confused, mixing up the Martelli and the Gozzini laws. In actual fact, the Martelli law disciplines immigration and redefines the status of the refugee and so would have had no effect on Martino at all. What, therefore, are Martino's memories? Why did he respond to the question regarding the differences between life in prison and life in the FPH with this rambling, confused discourse with weak associative connections, and memories that overlapped erratically? Martino himself provided more information about his state of health: "Dual personality. This means that you aren't you. [omissis] With this dual personality, one is OK, the other, well, the other makes you commit … I don't know, robberies, for example. I'm not happy here in the FPH. I don't have psychiatric pathologies to compare with paranoids, schizophrenics, maniacs". And in fact, he is not suffering from primary psychosis.

However, Martino provided another clue to his diagnosis when he reflects on his past and his first experience in a FPH in Aversa. "I was there under observation, I came from prison because I was in Favignana where I was doing manual work. Well, in their opinion I had a bit of mental illness. Caused by alcohol. I drank a bit in prison. Yep. I drank: half a liter of alcohol, wine or beer. All legal and above board, just that I overdid it. It's not the quarter of alcohol that you drink. It's that out of ignorance you try to see if you can get drunk. Ignorance leads to these sorts of things. Was I bored? Were we bored? No, don't think so. It's just you get yourself all revved up and challenge the alcohol to change you. But it takes years to figure out that it changes you. In fact it does, alcohol does: easy writing under the influence. When I read and I wasn't high anymore I'd rip up the letters and didn't send them. They were all about "bring me this", "do that for me". Alcohol is a damned nuisance that you've got to get in hand. I lost my mind to alcohol."

So here we have it. Martino's first experience with the FPH was due to alcohol abuse and the consequent psychic disturbances. Indeed, his addiction to alcohol during his early periods in prison is common to many, as emerged from the meta-analysis conducted in 2006 by Seena Fazel and colleagues[9] who found that the prevalence of alcohol abuse/addiction in male prisoners varies from 18% to 30%. At the time of writing, Martino was sixty-five years old and both his face and speech were scarred by alcohol abuse. He was clearly suffering from the effects of organic brain damage caused by this abuse, as evidenced by memory lapses, mental confusion and a tendency to confabulate.

The term *confabulate* has its origins in the early seventeenth century; it comes from the Latin verb *confabulari*, *con-*'together' + *fabulari* 'talk' (from *fabula* 'fable'). Carl Wernicke was the first to use it in the medical literature in the early 1900s. In psychiatric terms it is used to identify "a complex and probably non-unitary phenomenon which could represent a mechanism to preserve continuity of the sense of self in a context of cognitive deficits"[10]

Indeed, Martino's response to the opening question regarding his perception of the differences between life in prison and in the FPH, when he

[9] Fazel, S., Bains, P., & Doll, H. (2006). Substance abuse and dependence in prisoners: a systematic review. *Addiction (Abingdon, England)*, *101*(2), 181–191. https://doi.org/10.1111/j.1360-0443.2006.01316.x.

[10] Rossi, A. (2010). Confabulazione. Maj, M., Maggini, C., Siracusano, A. (eds.), *Lessico di Psicopatologia*, Il Pensiero Scientifico Editore. (our translation).

mentions the confusion in the FPH compared to the in prison, and starts to cite the Gozzini and Martelli laws, Vallanzasca, the protests, shows all the characteristics of confabulation.

> In 1901, Bonhoeffer distinguished the confabulation of embarrassment (later termed *momentary confabulation*) from spontaneous confabulation. Confabulation of embarrassment referred to fabricated memories that appeared to compensate for memory loss—in effect, the patient attempts to cover up an exposed *gap in memory*. In contrast, Bonhoeffer described spontaneous confabulation as exceeding the need to cover a memory deficit and often consisting of *fantastic* (grossly implausible) content.[11]

Martino would appear to resort to both these types of confabulation associated with his addiction to alcohol; indeed they are symptoms of a clinical psycho-organic condition known as Alcohol-related brain damage, which has been defined as "[…] an umbrella term that includes Wernicke-Korsakoff syndrome, alcohol-related dementia, and other forms of persistent alcohol-related cognitive impairment. Wernicke-Korsakoff syndrome is predominantly a thiamine deficiency state, whereas alcohol-related dementia is mainly a manifestation of alcohol-induced neurotoxicity. However, both may co-exist in the same individual, introducing substantial heterogeneity in their presentation".[12]

Wernicke's encephalopathy is a medical emergency. Without appropriate treatment, death ensues in 20% of cases while 75% of those who survive are left with permanent brain damage and memory loss (Korsakoff's Psychosis).[13]

Korsakoff himself attributed this condition principally to an abuse of alcohol accompanied by nutritional impoverishment (thiamine deficiency). Although he did not mention Wernicke's encephalopathy

[11] Chlebowski, S.M., Chung, C., Alao, A., Pies, R.W. (2009). Confabulation: A Bridge Between Neurology and Psychiatry? *Psychiatric Times*, *26*(6).

[12] Rao, R., & Draper, B. (2015). Alcohol-related brain damage in older people. *The lancet. Psychiatry*, *2*(8), 674–675. https://doi.org/10.1016/S2215-0366(15)00215-1, Vol. 2, 2015.

[13] Thomson, A. D., & Marshall, E. J. (2006). The natural history and pathophysiology of Wernicke's Encephalopathy and Korsakoff's Psychosis. *Alcohol and alcoholism (Oxford, Oxfordshire)*, *41*(2), 151–158. https://doi.org/10.1093/alcalc/agh249.

specifically, he did state that prodromic confusion and agitation usually precede this memory disorder, which is sometimes also accompanied by ophthalmoplegia, nystagmus, ataxia. He noted that "At first, during conversation with such a patient … [he or she] gives the impression of a person in complete possession of his [or her] faculties; he [she] reasons about everything perfectly well, draws correct deductions from premises, makes witty remarks, plays chess or a game of cards, in a word comports himself [herself] as a mentally sound person … [However], the patient constantly asks the same questions and repeats the same stories … may read the same page over and again sometimes for hours … is unable to remember those persons whom he [she] met only during the illness, for example, the attending physician or nurse."[14]

Memory of recent events is seriously compromised, as is the memory of events that occurred during the illness and, in some cases, even those in the past. In less severe cases, such as could be Martino's, under favorable conditions the person has a vague recollection of recent events, as the loss of memory is mainly related to thought processes. In some cases, the person has a full recollection of the event, but not of the time frame in which it occurred. Oliver Sacks described such a case in painstaking detail in the story of *the Lost Mariner* in his book, *The Man who Mistook his Wife for a Hat*.[15] Korsakoff noted that such patients "would tell of conversations which have never occurred, and so forth. [They] invent some fiction and constantly repeat it so that a peculiar delirium develops, rooted in false recollections (pseudo-reminiscences)".[16] They also tend to confuse memories of past events with impressions of the present, bringing up genuine recollections, but in the wrong context and time frame. He also remarked on "repetitive questionings, the extensive nature of the

[14] Victor, M., & Yakovlev, P. I. (1955). S.S. Korsakoff's psychic disorhic disorder in conjunction with peripheral neuritis; a translation of Korsakoff's original article with comments on the author and his contribution to clinical medicine. *Neurology, 5*(6), 394–406. https://doi.org/10.1212/wnl.5.6.394.

[15] Sacks, O. (1998). *The Man who mistook his wife for a Hat: and other clinical tales*. Simon and Schuster.

[16] Victor, M., & Yakovlev, P. I. (1955). S. S. Korsakoff's psychic disorder in conjunction with peripheral neuritis; a translation of Korsakoff's original article with brief comments on the author and his contributions to clinical medicine. *Neurology, 5*, 394–406. https://doi.org/10.1212/WNL.5.6.394.

retrograde memory loss, and a particular problem in remembering the temporal sequence of events, associated with severe disorientation in time."[17]

It would be interesting to know how Martino's recollections of the Gozzini and Martelli laws, the protests in prison, his encounters with Vallanzasca, took form in his mind. A clue to this might be his perception of the two laws while he was in prison. In a study published on the *Journal of Nervous and Mental Disorders* in 2003, Ingrid Candel and her colleagues investigated the involvement of the amygdala in the formation of flashbulb memories[18] in a group of patients with Korsakoff syndrome. Taken together with a similar study by Ikeda et al. (1998) on the memories of AD patients regarding the Kobe earthquake, it emerged that impairment of the amygdala affected recall of these emotionally charged events in these two groups.[19] [20] It is in fact well known that patients with the Korsakoff syndrome tend to suffer lesions of the mammillary bodies, the anterior section of the thalamus and the frontal lobes (Kopelman, 1995).[21] It is indeed possible that during the 1980s when he was in prison Martino was particularly and personally affected by the terms of the Gozzini law regulating permits, early releases and so on, with the result that he had a high emotive involvement with the subject, so thirty years later the question regarding the differences between prisons and FPH afforded him the opportunity to revive these memories.

During his ruminations on the question of the differences, Martino introduced another interesting element, simulation. He mentioned that in prison he had encountered individuals who simulated mental illnesses

[17] Kopelman, M. D. (1995). The Korsakoff syndrome. *The British Journal of Psychiatry, 166*(2), 154–173. https://doi.org/10.1192/bjp.166.2.154.

[18] The term used to indicate a type of memory resembling a highly vivid and detailed 'snapshot' of a moment in which a consequential, surprising and emotionally arousing item of news was learned.

[19] Candel, I., Jelicic, M., Merckelbach, H., & Wester, A. (2003). Korsakoff patients' memories of September 11, 2001. *The Journal of nervous and mental disease, 191*(4), 262–265. https://doi.org/10.1097/01.NMD.0000061142.82435.BC.

[20] Ikeda M, Mori E, Hirono N, et al. Amnestic people with Alzheimer's disease who remembered the Kobe earthquake. *British Journal of Psychiatry*. 1998;172(5):425–428. https://doi.org/10.1192/bjp.172.5.425.

[21] Kopelman, M. D. (1995). The Korsakoff syndrome. *The British Journal of Psychiatry, 166*(2), 154–173. https://doi.org/10.1192/bjp.166.2.154.

to obtain an acquittal and a transfer to the FPH for therapy, convinced that by so doing they would obtain an earlier release. Martino explained that prisoners will even go the whole hog and simulate suicide, to have thirty years in prison commuted into ten in the FPH. However, he pointed out that "… that's a mistake because there are extensions to make sure you don't get out after ten years. They extend your sentence like they did to me, fourteen extensions I got." His reasoning here appears coherent with what is known as twin-track confinement: detention in prison, therapy in FPH. It is possible to be transferred from prison to FPH, from one track to the other, but what usually happens is that a person suffering from a mental illness who has committed a crime is subjected to a course of therapy in the FPH that lasts longer than the prison sentence for that crime, due also to the extensions. There are many reasons judges opt to extend the inmate's period in the FPH: a difficult situation at home, or even a flat refusal from relatives to accommodate the inmate after the term of internment in the FPH is concluded, psychiatric services that are not adequate to assist in the outside world, the patient may not be completely recovered, delays in paperwork caused by incompetent lawyers. Domenico Casagrande, who was director of the Psychiatric Hospital of San Clemente, Venice, Italy until its closure in 1992, and was a member of the organizing committee of *Psichiatria Democratica,*[22] made the following statement in the movement's 2011 conference.

It is important to remember that people who end up in a FPH for a certain period of time often die in those institutions either because they don't have a family, or because their family doesn't want to have them in the home, considering them to be "mentally unsound" or "a danger to society". […]. By this I certainly do not mean to say that the patient shouldn't have to pay his debt to society for the crime he has committed, what I do mean is that the punishment has to be proportionate to the crime. I will go further: if a person has to be treated, he/she must have the

[22] *Psichiatria Democratica* is an Italian movement created by a group of psychiatrists, sociologists and social workers under direction of Franco Basaglia. The original committee consisted of Franca Basaglia, Franco Basaglia, Domenico Casagrande, Franco di Cecco, Tullio Fragiacomo, Vieri Marzi, Gian Franco Minguzzi, Piera Piatti, Agostino Pirella, Michele Risso, Lucio Schittar, Antonio Slavich. The movement called for radical changes in the practice and theory of psychiatry and was influential in promoting legislative reforms in this field.

same rights as any other person and should not, must not be subjected to a punishment such as the FPH, because being locked up in a FPH means to die each day, and being subjected to a punishment without end.

Strong words, denouncing the situation that the Parliamentary Commission of Inquiry[23] discovered in the FPHs and which led to the emanation of Law 81, May 30, 2014 that states "the duration of provisional or definitive custodial measures, including hospitalization in Residences for the Execution of Custodial Measures, shall not extend beyond the period established for imprisonment, taking into consideration the maximum statutory sentence applicable for the crime committed. The period of imprisonment will be determined on the base of article 278 of the Italian Penal Code." This law is intended to put an end to these cases of "life sentences without sentencing". Martino gave a perfect description of how the extensions work, "If they say to me, "Go and find a way of making your living outside of here", I'll go back to my town and I'll find somewhere to live and a job. Here it's difficult. I've been here in Rehab since the beginning of April. I've got a review on the 13th. My lawyer hasn't found any project or Rehab, when he does the judge will send me there. But the Social Services don't do anything right away, they'll let the extension expire." When I talked to him, he was at the Carmen Salpietro Rehabilitation Centre for the final probation period prior to his final review with the judge.

Summing up, Martino entered the prison system around 1973, and then was transferred to the FPH in Aversa for observation in 1976 when he was 29 years old; he attempted an escape and was returned to prison. Then, having obtained application of article 89 of the Italian penal code (diminished capacity), he was sent to a halfway house in Montelupo for six years and then to Barcellona Pozzo di Gotto, with various unsuccessful stays in work colonies and other rehabilitation centers, for a total of

[23] The Parliamentary Commission of Inquiry into the efficacy and efficiency of the National Health Service was instituted by the Italian Senate on July 30, 2008. Prof. Ignazio Marino was nominated President of the Commission. The final report was approved by the Commission on January 30, 2013 and included a section on the FPHs, including reports on unannounced visits (including Barcellona Pozzo di Gotto in June 2010) conducted by a group of politicians led by Prof. Marino in person. The findings of the Commission were instrumental to the closure of the FPH.

forty years spent in imprisonment and psychiatric institutions. Forty years, when his sentence in the 1970s was for 5 years and 6 months. However, he seems to have come to terms with his crimes and the life he has led, which he commented on quite positively, "Now all I want to do is to put the past behind me, because it's all experience and I need it. But I tell myself it wasn't a negative experience because I could have committed much more serious crimes than I did, as I was ignorant, not having had the benefit of culture from school. I haven't got a diploma, but I've learned plenty of lessons from life…".

He finished the interview returning to the original question, the difference between being a prisoner in jail and a patient in the FPH, "It's true that people with mental illnesses never get better, but I'm fine, why should I get ill? I've gotten over other people's pathologies by being a psychiatrist for them. I've got a certain background. Like now, I'm together with youngsters with schizophrenic and deliriant pathologies. It's not a dialogue between inmates, "Don't worry, I've got a pal who has a lot of land and we'll go and work there". This kind of conversation just doesn't exist in the FPH. Here there's the hate and the abandonment that there used to be in the mental asylums, because that is what these places are. They've gone back to being mental asylums."

Giancarlo: The Diagnosis and Involuntary Commitment (TSO)

Obstructing an Officer in His Line of Duty

I'm Giancarlo. I've been here for three and a half years. I'm here because I put up resistance during an involuntary commitment. What I did was involuntary. I never thought I'd do that. These people came to the house, I was taking a pill each day and I wanted to stop taking them because I wanted out of this situation. That's all there was to it, but the director ordered this involuntary commitment and all those people came. Ambulances, traffic police, national police, not even Totò Riina got such a turnout. At that point I came down, saw all those people, I resisted them, see, because I wanted to rebel and because they've been doing this to me for years, in the street, wherever. Only because the judge, the mayor, two doctors, signed. That's what it takes to start the process. They capture you like an animal. It makes you look bad; people look at you askance after they see you being taken away like that. They shoot drugs into you while you're lying on the ground, sometimes I wake up weeks later with a drip in my arm.

I was in therapy because I'd had a fight with two guys. The carabinieri arrived and took me to the barracks, they beat me up then when they saw what they'd done they took me to the A&E ward. I was completely immobile, they had kicked me everywhere with their pointed shoes, and when I say everywhere I mean everywhere, my balls, my face. I complained to the doctor about this and he pushed me onto the ground and put handcuffs on me and kicked me some more. At that point they called a lady psychiatrist who saw that I was furious because of what she said to me. She said I wasn't well. That was the first time I was hospitalized. After that they've never let me be. Whatever the doctor said ended up in an involuntary commitment and it's happened over and over again. Because I fought against it, I wanted to put an end to this.

My Diagnosis

They say I'm bipolar. They say I go from one phase to another without realizing it. But it's not true. It's my character, it's the way I am. If I have to tell you to f**k off, I'll tell you to your face; if not, I won't. The psychiatrists have done this to justify all what has happened, they had to write something. They've never given me a pension. They've granted me a disability of just 60%. I've been here for three and a half years; I was only supposed to do two. They gave me an extra year and a half because in the Department of Mental Health they washed their hands of me because according to them I don't follow the therapy and they could have problems. And so here I am in the FPH, the safest place they could put me. Don't know if it's safest for me or for them. It's certainly the safest option for them. Because if I could get out, I would … But there's no rhyme or reason to what they say. Even the social worker said, "but how is he supposed to follow the therapy here? This is the question. Is there any hope the situation will change?".

What is an FPH? You want to know what I think? Some say it's a human refuse dump, a lot of people say that, but not the doctor. In my opinion, from what I've seen here and on television, you can't do without them. I'll say that loud and clear. But without the drugs. There are people who have to be here, people you couldn't put in prison or in a rehab center to serve their sentence. Here they are treated, but there should be a project for these people, there should be more psychologists, more staff, not just one psychiatrist.

I feel the need for treatment, but who doesn't these days? Sometimes, yes, but sometimes no! I'm fine with the pill and a half that I take, because there's nothing they haven't done to me… three injections a day. I know I have these mood swings, but it's their fault. I can get on with anyone and everyone, but I can't stand arrogance and bullying. It happened when I was a kid as well, when I wasn't mad. Even when no one said I was mad, I was like this. Only my mother maintained I was mad. Once, when I said I that I'd been mad for the past twelve months, she said, "no, you've always been like that". There are people much worse off than I am. They could put me in a rehab center. I've been in Padre Pippo's Halfway House about fifteen times. It's not bad there, but not for ever…

A typical day in the FPH: you do something in your cell, wash some clothes, watch television. I listen to something on my player, I like music, I've been in a lot of bands in the past. I've got a poem about these things, it's called *Chains*. It's all about these places.

I used to write, I sing and I compose, I can play an instrument too. But I'm not a musician. I'd like to be, though. If I get out of here, I know someone I can go make music with.

I was born in Naples, but I lived in Puglia for a long time and now I'm Sicilian. I did a month and a half inside in Taranto for hashish. I came here straight from Taranto after being shut up in a bunker for eleven days where there was nothing. There was a toilet and a shower, no windows. It was all dark, no light, disgusting. They didn't even come to clean. Eleven days without food in Taranto. They had to validate the arrest. They couldn't arrest me because I'd committed the offense during the involuntary commitment, and so for the law I was of unsound mind. I couldn't be charged, but they arrested me anyway. Then I was acquitted. Acquitted for insanity. And they didn't even give me 80% disability so I could get a pension! That's abuse!

The Fine Line Between Reason and Madness

You want to know what I think of mental illness? What can I say? Mental illness is a bit more when one ... there's a fine line between reason and madness, so fine that you're not even aware of it and you can go from one to the other without realizing.

Maybe the people you're with realize it, but then, they can go from one to the other too, and you realize that when they are out of their mind. There are many types of illness, and various forms of mental illness. I know mine, and here I've come across lots of others. Once I looked at this person, then said something to him and I ended up with a punch in the teeth. I got three stitches. They almost killed me here, I was in a coma for three days, they tried to strangle me in my sleep. Why? How should I know? I never found out. Now I feel safe, things are better, at that time I didn't know people. They put me in that room. Now I get on fine with my neighbors.

Danger to the public? Here you see folk who can hardly put one foot in front of the other. I can't see them being much of a danger to the public. It's an abuse of power, it's the law that discriminates against a person and leaves them here to rot. Then there are others who should be here, people here who have committed real crimes, *mafiosi*, people who have killed their father, or their mother. In these cases, it's right that they should be labelled as being a danger to the public, but it should diminish over time. It can't always be the same degree of danger. There are cases of people who have been treated and stabilized but can't leave because they are still considered to be a danger to the public. There's a law that says that if you don't leave here and go first to a rehab center, they can't say you are no longer a danger to society. It can take years to get the judge to state you aren't a danger anymore. There are people who have never managed this. They just stay here, in bed. After years and years, they die here, skin and bone. Lots of medicine, lots, every day.

On television you see these activists making a fuss about dolphins, dogs, but no one does that for the people in here.

In the future, if they give me the time, there are a lot of things I'd like to do. I'm thirty-six years old, I could do lots, but they have to give me time. And another chance. After all, I have never committed a theft, and I've never pushed drugs. I think they'll give me another chance. I've got a family, a daughter. She's fifteen now, she sings too, she's starting to write her first songs, she studies languages in high school. She's bright and I'd love to see her. I haven't seen her in five years. These would be the best years to be with her. Being shut in here and only being able to talk to her on the phone, that's grim.

Reflections on Giancarlo's Interview

"They say I'm *bi-polar*". This is how Giancarlo, a thirty-seven-year-old Neapolitan, who appeared rather cunning and infantile in his approach, labelled himself in the interview. He doesn't know much about bipolar disorders and cares even less, what concerned him—he says—are the effects: based on this diagnosis, psychiatrists ordered numerous involuntary commitments because he was refusing treatment, culminating in the final episode when Giancarlo *obstructed an officer in the course of his duty*. Together with the psychiatrist's diagnosis, this resulted in the charges against him being dropped and his hospitalization in the FPH.

We know very little of Giancarlo's psychopathology, all he says is that "they say I go from one phase to another without realizing it. But it's not true. It's my character, it's the way I am. If I have to tell you to f**k off, I'll tell you to your face; if I don't, I won't." Then he added, and his tone became more serious, "I feel the need for treatment, but who doesn't these days? Sometimes, yes, but sometimes no! I'm fine with the pill and a half (Tolep) that I take, because in the past there's nothing they haven't done to me… three injections a day. I know I have these *mood swings*, but it's their fault. I can get on with anyone and everyone, but I can't stand arrogance and bullying. It happened when I was a kid as well, when I wasn't mad. Even when no one said *I was mad*, I was like this. Only my mother maintained I was mad. Once, when I said I that *I'd been mad for* *the past twelve months*, she said, "*no, you've always been like that*". At that point, we both laughed a bit, to take the edge off his words.

In Giancarlo's brief description of his mental state there is evidence of the mood swings, from the maniacal to the depressive, together with impulsive and reactive features vis-à-vis the Other (in the Lacanian sense of the term) that characterize the disturbance. What I found interesting in his account is the operational significance he attributes to the diagnosis, which provides the opportunity to formulate some considerations regarding the value of diagnosis in psychiatry. "The psychiatrists have done this to justify all what has happened, they had to write something. They've never given me a pension. They've granted me a disability of just 60%." Giancarlo felt that this diagnosis of a bipolar disturbance wasn't finalized in a real course of treatment, nor did it provide him with any economic benefits (a disability pension); in his view, it was simply a justification for the involuntary commitments he had been subjected to.

Ergo, for Giancarlo these involuntary commitments were not, in sé, a treatment "beyond the limit of the mental illness" or a treatment that has to be obligatory due to the irreducible and compulsive nature of the illness that the patient himself has difficulty in recognizing. This has been clearly explained by Dr. Pietro Pellegrini Director of the Mental Health Unit of the Local Health Authority of Parma:

Usually, treatment of mental disturbances is voluntary, and based on consensus. Why, then, are involuntary commitments used? Certain mental disturbances can cause a lack of awareness of the illness and patients may refuse the urgent treatment necessary because their representations and ability to evaluate situations have been severely compromised by the illness. Involuntary commitment is therefore the last, extreme resource to safeguard the right to health of a person suffering from a grave psychic pathology of which they are not aware. It is performed in the public interest not as a "social defense mechanism" but rather to restore the patient to their place in society. There must always be an attempt to obtain the consensus of the person involved.

Under Italian law,[24] three main conditions must be present before an involuntary commitment can be executed: evident signs of a mental dis-

[24] Article 34, Law 833/78.

turbance that requires immediate therapeutic treatment; the person refuses the therapeutic treatment (the refusal is closely related to the disturbed mental state); the treatment can only be administered on hospital premises.

Giancarlo's perception of the involuntary commitment is limited to the coercive element and not to the treatment. Indeed, this occurs in many cases, not only Giancarlo's. Why is this? Of course, no patient undergoing an involuntary commitment procedure is in a state to recognize the treatment aspect, particularly if restraint is being used. However, if after hospitalization the patient accepts the treatment and it produces positive results, they can recognize that the involuntary commitment was indeed the beginning, the *first step of the cure*. This however is not the case with Giancarlo who remembers only the coercive aspect, the attempt to curb the condition that is rendering him a danger to society.

There is a typically *anti-psychiatry* flavor to the comments Giancarlo made during his interview; he comes across as a Prometheus Chained, a titan condemned to suffer involuntary commitments, chained to the rock of psychiatry by a psychiatric diagnosis and consequent institutionalization of the treatment, ordered by a nebulous being, an undefined sovereign-or psychiatrist-Zeus. It is no coincidence that Giancarlo wrote and sang a video-poem about chains, to describe the state of many psychiatric patients, condemned to being abandoned to their fate and coercive treatments.

Chains
Chains for those
who are the brunt of absurd apathy
rearing majestic walls
across their path.

Chains for those
Who although they are free
Are slaves to the system
And its perpetual presumptions
Of power and injustice.

And while everything flows
Around me swiftly
And the past becomes the present
And the present becomes the future
I find myself behind bars
chained to rocks.
I await the rising of the sun.
Long silences.
White rooms
Stained by the passing of passers-by.
Grey faces, eyes veiled with crystal tears
That fall to the floor with a sweet sound
To chant their lament
While the wind beats against the windows
as if trying to get in to defend us
against those shadows at the door
with their gloves and white coats
that remind you of suffering.

Like pointed awls
The words spoken in those moments
And with false smiles
Poison our dreams
And cut like knives.
Knives that do not care
And wound your soul.

But wait if you want.
I am what you want me to be.
You'll have to wait awhile.
This is pure torment! Woman!

Don't hate me if this is not the time
For love.
Don't chase me if I run away from this reality.
You can't catch me.
What do you know of the pain I feel?
Only chains
For the man who fights.

The imagery of the *tears of crystal* falling to the floor and creating a *sweet sound*, and the *wind beating against the windows* as if trying to get in to defend the patients from the *shadows at the door* is particularly evocative. He uses these words to represent the suffering of psychiatric patients sent to the Psychiatric Diagnosis and Care Service, many of whom remain locked in these institutions for years, marked by a more or less adequate diagnosis. These patients are not always fortunate enough to meet psychiatrists and health workers who are willing to listen.

Much of what Giancarlo says about his diagnosis, or his *diagnosis in psychiatry* is reflected in an article written by Mario Colucci, an Italian psychiatrist and psychoanalyst working in the Mental Health Department in Trieste. Colucci is on the editorial board of *Aut Aut*, an Italian quarterly publication dealing with philosophy and the human sciences; in a special edition dedicated to *The diagnosis in psychiatry*, he describes the effect of labelling in psychiatric diagnosis in an article entitled *Fabrizio, with one zed. A critique of diagnostic reasoning.* Fabrizio, the patient described in the article, is sectioned in a PDCS, in a closed ward, and has been diagnosed as a schizophrenic, or, as the health workers would have it, *schizzophrenic* (a play on the Italian *schizzato*, slang for weirdo, lunatic). He is often constrained, tied to his bed because he is "unmanageable". Early on in his career Colucci had asked why Fabrizio was often constrained, and the answer he received, almost derisively, was "because he is a *schizzophrenic*!" The diagnosis defines the person and the treatment he receives.

Colucci wrote, "The diagnosis functions as an absolute, a definitive judgement, almost to underline the irrefutable fact of the illness as opposed to the chaos of opinions: an ancient torment that springs from the eternal dissatisfaction with an unacknowledged scientific charter. According to Michel Foucault, the root of the problem is the lack of a solid foundation for its corpus of knowledge; it can be said that while anatomy is the keystone of modern medicine, psychiatry has searched in vain for the source of its knowledge in the morgues. Knowledge of the mind is not to be constructed on information from dissected bodies; warm, live and recalcitrant bodies are needed for this, to be subdued in the asylums [...]. This is the reason that psychiatry, with its dual therapeutic and biopolitical vocation, attempts to adopt an inflexible criterion of inclusion/exclusion with which it can confirm the presence or absence of madness from the first observation and so to take a black and white decision regarding a course of treatment in an institution, or incarceration: in other words, to decide whether the person involved should walk away free or be remanded into custody. The issue is to reach an absolute rather than a differential diagnosis, that is, not to distinguish between the various forms of madness—along the lines of a Kraepelinian treatise—but to establish, without the shadow of a doubt, the presence or absence of madness."

Mario Colucci's opinion brings to mind Giancarlo's words about *being mad*, "It happened when I was a kid as well, when I wasn't mad. Even when no one said *I was mad*, I was like this. Only my mother maintained I was mad. Once, when I said I that *I'd been mad for the past twelve months*, she said, "*no, you've always been like that*"."

What was really important to Giancarlo, more than the diagnosis of "bipolar disorder" which as far as he was concerned is just the same as any other, was being called mad by a third party, in this case his mother, who drew the line between being sound of mind and madness, and who considered that her son had always been mad. Giancarlo's story, which has many points in common with that of *Fabrizio, with one 'z'*, underlines the importance of a *definitive diagnosis*. It has defined Giancarlo's destiny. Every sign of a deficit, each refusal to follow the treatment prescribed, finishes in an involuntary commitment. In this particular case, as he "obstructed an officer in the course of executing the involuntary commitment" he ended up in the FPH, for a course of treatment and to guarantee public safety.

Roberto Beneduce, anthropologist and ethno-psychiatrist, provided an interesting point of view regarding diagnosis in psychiatry that throws light on what Giancarlo tried to convey in his story.

> Psychiatric diagnosis, on the contrary, seems to want to refute uncertainty: sometimes its routine resembles a crystal violently plunged into the body of experience, with the effect of shattering "human temporality" and putting an end to the infinite process of interpretation. Notwithstanding this, its guidelines are quite different, often characterized by resigned pragmatism: it is used according to what is required at the time (a medical certificate, a patient's request to reply to some institution), and nobody really

> believes what is written. However, one of the most paradoxical profiles of psychiatric diagnosis originates from the strange conjunction between its structural epistemological weakness on the one hand, and its performative power on the other. A psychiatric diagnosis can affect one's right to continue as a parent, to work in a specific environment, obtain refugee status in another country; one's very life can depend on it. The "stigmatization" that sometimes surrounds a psychiatric diagnosis is merely the better-known expression of a deep and ambiguous undercurrent, punctuated by disorganized procedures in the interstices of which subjectivity reigns supreme and determines the destiny of the unfortunate patient.[25]

Psychiatric diagnosis is indeed performative. A person suffering from a bipolar disorder (in this case) reacts badly to an officer trying to execute an involuntary commitment, considered necessary as the person involved is psychopathic and has not followed his course of treatment—the person is immediately sent to the FPH. His future is marked out. As Beneduce says, his destiny has been determined. Art. 341 bis of the Italian Penal Code establishes that obstructing an officer in the execution of his duty is punishable by up to three years imprisonment. Giancarlo said that he had been given two years that was extended by eighteen months as the Department of Mental Health had declined to accept him due to the fact that he did not follow the prescribed course of treatment. "And so here I am in the FPH, the safest place they could put me. Don't know if it's safest for me or for them. It's certainly the safest option for them." This raises the question of *safety*, who has to feel safe? The person with the illness or society?

Talking about *what is mental illness?* Giancarlo went back to the question of the demarcation between sanity and madness. He said, "Mental illness is a bit more when one … there's a fine line between reason and madness, so fine that you're not even aware of it and you can go from one to the other without realizing. Maybe the people you're with realize it, but then, they can go from one to the other too, and you realize it only when they are out of their mind." The American psychiatrist Allen Frances expands on the theme of the *fine line between reason and madness* in his book *Saving Normal* regarding the diagnostic methodology of the various

[25] Beneduce, R. (2013). Illusioni e Violenza della diagnosi psichiatrica. *Aut Aut 357*, La diagnosi in psichiatria. 187–211 (our translation).

DSMs (Diagnostic and Statistical Manual of Mental Disorders). Dr. Frances chaired the American Psychiatric Association task force overseeing the development and revision of the fourth edition of the DSM but found himself in disaccord with his colleagues of the task force that worked on the fifth edition, claiming that it lowered the threshold for many diagnoses, resulting in an inflation of mental disorders diagnosed in the population and a corresponding increase in the consumption of anti-psychotic medication. His reasoning is based on the concepts of normality and pathology, and his critique is aimed at those colleagues who drew up a statistical and diagnostic manual that tipped the balance toward pathology.

In the preface to his book, he clarified that "My nightmare scenario is that some people will do a selective reading and draw the completely incorrect and unintended conclusion that I am against psychiatric diagnosis and treatment," and went on to say "My hope is to simultaneously serve two purposes—first to alert people who don't need treatment to avoid it, but equally to encourage those who do need treatment to seek it out and to stick with it. My critique is directed only against the excesses of psychiatry, not its heart or soul. "Saving normal" and "saving psychiatry" are really two sides of the very same coin."[26]

In *Essentials of psychiatric diagnosis: responding to the challenge of DSM-5,* he further clarified his position regarding psychiatric diagnosis: "Done well, psychiatric diagnosis leads to appropriate treatment and a good chance for cure or at least substantial improvement. Done poorly, psychiatric diagnosis leads to a nightmare of harmful treatments, unnecessary stigma, missed opportunities, reduced expectations, and negative self-fulfilling prophecies."[27] He pointed out that in psychiatry, diagnosis is based on subjective judgements that are inescapably fallible, and so should be constantly verified as the practitioner builds his relationship with the patient and observes the development of the disorder.

[26] Frances, A. (2013). *Saving normal: An insider's revolt against out-of-control psychiatric diagnosis, DSM-5, Big Pharma, and the medicalization of ordinary life.* William Morrow & Co. (Preface).

[27] Frances, A. (2013). *Essentials of psychiatric diagnosis: Responding to the challenge of DSM-5®* (Revised ed.). Guilford Press.

In synthesis, the interview with Giancarlo revolves around the question of psychiatric diagnosis. It is clear from his comment, "They say I'm bipolar", that he doesn't recognize that he has this illness; *they* made this diagnosis, *they* called him bipolar, it isn't *his* diagnosis. What would *his* diagnosis have been if he had been able to contribute to it? Not a diagnosis that someone else has stuck on him like a label, *his* personal diagnosis. Indeed, it takes two to make a diagnosis, the observer (the clinician) and the observed (the patient). The Greek etymology of the term is *knowledge through observation* and traditionally, diagnosis has been defined as the art of identifying a disease from its signs and symptoms. Attributing a name to the clinical phenomenon, to the collection of signs, symptoms and behavior helps to identify a course of treatment that can halt the pathogenesis.

Formerly, few diagnostic tests were available to assist the physician, who depended on the patient's medical history, observation, and examination. Now diagnostic tools such as Computed Axial Tomography (CAT) scans, Nuclear Magnetic Resonance (NMR), Single-photon Emission Computerized Tomography (SPECT), Positron Emission Tomography (PET), are frequently used in medicine to identify signs and symptoms, contributing additional data to the diagnostic process. Psychiatry attempts to emulate classical medicine to construct a bio-medical model of mental illness, but without the support of diagnostic tools. Recently however, for certain diagnoses, psychiatry is approaching the level of knowledge of medicine that uses blood tests, neuroimaging, and genetic markers to confirm the indications provided by signs and symptoms. And the various editions of the DSM (DSM-1, 1952, 128 pages, 106 diagnoses—DSM-5, 2013, 947 pages, more than 300 diagnoses) represent a bio-medical attempt to provide a catalogue of mental disorders. The atheoretic nature and the universality of the presentation of the structure of each disorder renders the DSM a valid research tool. As Giuseppe Sabucco and Sergio Carfi wrote in their article, *L'odore della diagnosi* (The odour of the diagnosis), it is possible to catalogue all the world's mental disorders on the basis of their overlapping characteristics as found in the DSM: "The behavior of a confirmed schizophrenic will not differ substantially from another unfortunate who lives meridians away. The structure of a mental disorder, at least in the extreme forms, is relatively independent of the geographical, historical and cultural environment in which it develops. Vice versa, the identity of this same mental disorder is strengthened due to the universality of the presentation of its structure."[28]

This cultural operation of cataloguing mental disorders focusses on the disorders rather than on the people afflicted by them. A person who has been diagnosed as bipolar can have the same signs and symptoms as another person affected by this disorder, but that does not mean to say that they are the same. They will have different experiences, different working conditions, different friends and ways of interacting with them, different projects for the future.

Just like the DSM, the psychiatric institutions collaborate in a process of de-subjectification. Take involuntary commitment, for example. This can be experienced as a loss of subjectivity. Someone else, a doctor, equipped with all the necessary knowledge, takes your decisions for you. They decide whether the psychopathological crisis is severe enough to merit urgent treatment; you protest, say that that there is nothing wrong with you but the doctor considers that your objections are dictated by the gravity of the illness and so they act as guarantor and organize the involuntary commitment. It will take a good psychiatrist and a course of appropriate treatment for you to regain your sense of subjectivity, characterized by an awareness of the mental illness, acceptance of the treatment and a desire to change the status quo.

From what he has told us, it is evident that Giancarlo still has a negative view of the diagnosis because it obliges him to follow a course of treatment he does not want. But what would a positive view of a diagnosis be, a diagnosis that the person accepts, to the point of becoming part and parcel of their being, and which they describe as being a good diagnosis that they believe will lead to a successful course of treatment?

[28] Sabucco, G. & Carfi, S. (1999). L'Odore della Diagnosi. *Quaderni di Psichiatria pratica*, October 1999, a review published by the hospital of Melegnano.

Matteo: The Monster in the Medicine

You Get Up, Talk and Have a Fag

An FPH is a place where *a person exceeds a certain limit in understanding society*, where he can make good progress in society. You do your best, but maybe you overdo it. This is a place where they hold the prisoner back to slow him down, *to calm down his thoughts, clear his head*, maybe to bring him down to earth because he could rub someone up the wrong way. In Calabria they say, "It's always the same folk that eat". They do these things to take your dignity away.

The FPH is a *prison* because just like you take *medicine* here, you take it in prison, in a psychiatric ward, in involuntary commitment. This is when they keep you under observation. It doesn't need to be a year of suffering, the sentence that you have to do. They shouldn't take your shoelaces away: you look at a person and you put your trust in them because if you don't provoke a person …It's not that you ask for the moon and they have to give it you. You ask for what you need. Do your bit: me as a prisoner, you as a guard. You've no right to lay your hands on me.

The FPH is a place. Unfortunately, there are families that can't keep their relative at home, they can't deal with the situation, they might *self-harm*, do themselves an injury. Here people are taken care of, they're dressed well, they're calm, maybe when they see a guard they see a footballer, they fantasize, they see God, some think, some talk in one way, some in another. I don't know what else to say about the FPH. I don't know why they built them. I've seen lots of people coming and going here. I've seen people coming in with shiny, doll-like faces, baby-faces, and leaving deformed like *monsters*, after being treated here. That's not treatment. That's destroying people. Maybe you've treated their character problems or their moods, ok. But this torment you see in their faces, the dark circles under their eyes, you've made them suffer, you've annihilated them… that's not right at all. Prison in itself is a torment for the prisoner. Sleeping in a bed, losing your dignity. Look, for example, I'm a male. I'm not homosexual, I'm the way Nature intended us to be. If I think about seeing a woman here in front of me, paying her a compliment all the while with the fear that one of the guards could punch me; dignity is the worst thing in life. This is a bad thing that happens in these institutes. This is just me letting off steam. I'm twenty-one. This is how I see it. I had a girlfriend. We were engaged. I should have a three-year-old baby now. We lived together for a year and a half. My girlfriend had an abortion at the second month because my parents didn't want to take on the family. I should have been OK by now.

My days here? That's easy. You get up, you talk, you have a fag. I've been here before so there are people here I've already met. Some are quite decent and I chat with them because I see that it's OK to talk to them. You drink a coffee and pass the time of day. They offer you a bit of chocolate.

Mental Illness? Envy is at the Bottom of It

When we're kids, we're all the same. At eight years old, we're all the same. Maybe we all start smoking at the same time. But then someone's better off and someone else is poorer, someone gets a motorbike and starts *taking the mickey*, "I've got a motorbike and you're still hoofing it". Then you start growing up and you start doing your own thing; you get your own back on the guy with the motorbike, and not only on him. Maybe you get too much of a taste for it and overdo it; then you risk being left on your own. The moment these guys realize that you're watching them, they cut you off and push you into a form of depression because they start mocking you, "no, but you're like that", "things are this way, but you're that way"…sadly that's the way the world is…

My problem health-wise is to get a permanent job, so I can work and get myself back into society on my own. I'm trying, but unfortunately these places … when they see your medical records and what you've been through, when they see I've been in prison twice and twice in an FPH… I need a stroke of luck. My life is tougher now. If once a girl might have looked at me with a bit of respect, she wouldn't now. Eh, the FPH is no picnic, and the medicine makes it *worse*. And to make things worse, now it's hot.

My hopes for the future, I want to have a family. To have sincerity in the family, *to banish envy*, to not ruin a friend, not leave him in a mess just to get something for myself.

Reflections on Matteo's Interview

Matteo is a young man, just twenty-one years old. He came to the FPH in Barcellona from the prison in Reggio Calabria for psychiatric observation after trying to hang himself. This is the reason why he was not allowed to have his shoestrings, which he felt was an injustice, "They shouldn't take your shoelaces away: you look at a person and you put your trust in them because if you don't provoke a person …It's not that you ask for the moon and they have to give it you. You ask for what you need. Do your bit: me as a prisoner, you as a guard. You've no right to lay your hands on me.". He also complained that he had been beaten up in prison (I'm here because I accused the guard in charge, he slapped me, threw a stool at me", "the officers took photographs of me"). Very likely there was a brawl, after which Matteo probably filed a complaint. But this was not the reason he was placed under observation as he would have had us believe, the real reason was the attempted suicide, following which the prison authorities needed to understand the state of the prisoner's psychic health.

Matteo's childhood and early life was scarred by traumatic events: his father, who was involved in the 'Ndrangheta, committed suicide by jumping off a bridge probably while the boy was watching; his mother abandoned him by *declaring him to be a drug addict so the Social Services would lock him up*. He spoke very little about his crime which would appear to be drug related. He has always been institutionalized, *kidnapped* by the Social Services and put in a rehabilitation center first, then in a prison for having committed some misdemeanors, winding up finally in the FPH. In the absence of his parents, the institutions stepped in with treatment.

How does Matteo see the FPH?

> "An FPH is a place where *a person exceeds a certain limit in understanding society*, where he can make good progress in society. You do your best, but maybe you overdo it. This is a place where they hold the prisoner back to slow him down, *to calm down his thoughts, clear his head*, maybe to bring him down to earth because he could rub someone up the wrong way. In Calabria they say, "It's always the same folk that eat". They do these things to take your dignity away.
>
> The FPH is a prison because just like you take medicine here, you take it in prison, in a psychiatric ward, in involuntary commitment. This is when they keep you under observation. It doesn't need to be a year of suffering, the sentence that you have to do.

Matteo likens the FPH to prison, which has positive connotations for him as it helps people *to understand society, calm down thoughts*. A reflective function, therefore, as well as a restraining function that Matteo describes as "bringing him down to earth because he could rub someone up the wrong way". Here he is using the term *bringing down to earth* in two senses, i.e. in the first place, indicating how medicine is used to stabilize moods or sedate an explosion of rage, and the restraining nature of the place itself, and in the second place, there is the sense of diminishing the person, a lowering of height, a taking away of dignity, limits that are crossed. This has to do with the world of organized crime, with those who control the territory and its dynamics. "In Calabria they say, 'It's always the same folk that eat'. They do these things to take your dignity away". The FPH and the institution that Matteo has in mind is not closely linked to the State, but he sees it as being used by the powers that be in organized crime to get their own back or settle outstanding scores.

When talking about the treatments in the FPH, Matteo uses a neologism, *smostratura*,[29] to describe the effect of the anti-psychotics on the inmates. The term comes from *mostro*, monster and the verb, *smostrare*, to put into bad shape, to make someone look like a monster. "I've seen lots of people coming and going here. I've seen people coming in with shiny, doll-like faces, baby-faces, and leaving looking like *monsters*, after being treated here. That's not treatment. That's destroying people. Maybe you've

---

[29] Trifone P. (1996). Il linguaggio dei giovani di Pescara. *Contributi di Filologia dell'Italia Mediana.* X. 231–255.

treated their character problems or their moods, ok. But this torment you see in their faces, the dark circles under their eyes, you've made them suffer, you've annihilated them…"

In Matteo's perception, people arrive in the FPH with *shiny, doll-like faces*, transmitting a sort of innocence and purity notwithstanding the fact that they have committed a crime, in some cases a terrible crime. Then they come to the FPH and what happens? They are treated with anti-psychotics, they suffer, their suffering is there to be seen on their faces in the dark circles under their eyes, they die, in other words, they are left in bad shape. But who is the monster here? Monsters, in the fables of the nineteenth century, were not magical beings but humans who had undergone a transformation. There is always a case of redemption in these tales, and where there is a monster, the redemption takes the form of reversing the monster back into a human being.

The fables recounted by the brothers Jacob and Wilhelm Grimm provide examples of this.

The *Frog Prince* is the story of a frog that helped a princess. In exchange for finding her gold ball that she had lost in a pond, she promised to love him and keep him with her. She kept her promise with the help of her father, thus enabling the frog to change into a prince with laughing eyes and to marry the princess.

One of the best-known fables, *Little Red Riding Hood*, tells the story of a little girl in a red cape who crosses a dark wood to take a gift of food to her bedridden grandmother. The wolf, despite having eaten the grandmother, is not considered to be a monster as there is no redemption or transformation involved.

On the other hand, *The singing, springing lark*, the story of a girl who asks her father to bring her a lark back from his travels, has many transformations. To obtain the lark, the father has to promise a lion that he will send him the first person who comes to welcome him on his return to his castle. The first person is his beloved daughter, who willingly goes to maintain her father's promise. The lion turns out to be a prince after sundown and they marry, living happily until the girl wants to take him home to meet her family. A ray of light transforms the prince into a dove for seven years, but the girl follows him and, after many trials and misfortunes, manages to help him transform back into human form.

Jack my Hedgehog tells the story of a farmer and his wife who were childless; the farmer, exasperated, swore that he would father a child, be it only a hedgehog. Shortly after, much to his chagrin, his wife gave birth to a monstrous being, half human, half hedgehog, they called Jack my Hedgehog. Jack, aware of his father's displeasure, rode off to the woods on the back of a cockerel with a herd of pigs and a set of bagpipes. There he lived contentedly until he encountered a king who had lost his way. As in the story of the singing lark, Jack extorted a promise from the king to give him the first being that greeted the king on his return home. This he obtained, but the king deceived him. He then encountered another king and repeated the process. This time however, the king honored his promise and gave his daughter in marriage to Jack, who, by burning his spines, transformed into a complete human being.

The Donkey is a tale with a similar plot. The king and queen were rich and had everything they wanted except a child; the queen lamented this day and night, declaring that she was like a barren field where nothing grows. Finally, her prayers were answered, she fell pregnant, but gave birth to a donkey. His parents, the king and queen, rejected him, but he found shelter in the castle of a neighboring king who gave him his daughter in marriage. On their wedding night, the donkey shed his skin and was transformed into a handsome man.

Fables, then, are stories populated with anthropomorphic characters that contain a moral. They were an easily understandable medium for communicating moral teachings to children and adults alike. They usually contain an element of guilt, as can be seen in *The Donkey* and *Jack my Hedgehog*; in both these fables there is the implication that there must be a reason that the offspring born to these parents were animal (or partly animal) and not human. It is indeed only implied, the fable itself does not provide an explanation.

Iron Hans is the tale of a monster, "a wild man whose body was brown like rusty iron, and whose hair hung over his face down to his knees" who is released from a spell by the love and faithfulness of a young prince and so recovers his human form and earthly possessions.

Many psychoanalysts recommend reading fables to children to help them face their fears, both their intimate demons and monsters in the external world, as in these tales the monster never triumphs, but is domesticated or transformed by goodness. They contain awareness of evil, the difficulties we encounter in life, and the most important relationships. These therapeutic connotations make fables ideal for use in rehabilitation of psychoses, as a narrative truth onto which the psychotic can project his/her difficulties. The psychotic thought process follows the logic of the omnipotent and magical compensatory thought, which is part of the structure of the fable designed to obtain an immediate emotive participation. I came across an example of this with one of my patients, who suffers from a grave case of paranoid schizophrenia with delusions of persecution despite the medication he takes. One day he said to me, "I felt the bogeyman that's inside me, twisting and turning—it was an officer of the New York Police Department". Accepting that we have a bogeyman inside may refer to an imaginary monster which is tormenting us and with whom we have to struggle to overcome.

The imagery of the monster is also present in art.

In his second rendering of the *Sacrifice of Isaac* (1603), Caravaggio depicts Isaac's expression as twisted, deformed by anguish, the fear of death.

Diego Velasquez frequently included persons affected by dwarfism in his paintings of court life (as in his 1656 masterpiece *Las Meninas*), so endowing this condition with a certain dignity. Goya's aquatint of circa 1799, the *Sleep of Reason produces Monsters*, centers on the sleeping figure of a man, surrounded by hordes of monstrous nocturnal bird and bat-like creatures, and a diabolic cat crouching in a sphinx-like position, staring at the observer. As the title suggests, these creatures are the product of the man's mind.

"Imagination abandoned by reason produces impossible monsters; together with imagination, reason is the mother of the arts and source of wonders". According to Goya, imagination is the foundation of all creation. But if our imagination is allowed to rove uncontrolled without the support of reason it leads to monsters and other non-existent elements; if on the other hand, reason and imagination are united in an intimate alliance of rules and genius, an immensely powerful tool is created.

Another important work of art, *The Nightmare* by Johann Heinrich Fuseli (1791), depicts a monster, an incubus, crouched on the body of a sleeping woman, with the disembodied head of a blind horse in the background. According to Germanic folklore, such demons possessed the spirits of people who slept alone and so this depiction reflects the personification of the woman's nightmare.

Deformed faces bring to mind the works of Max Ernst (1891–1976), one of the leading exponents of the surrealism movement, the portraits painted by Francis Bacon (1909–1992), and the graffiti by Jean-Michel Basquiat (1960–1988).

Matteo perceives medication as a substance that can transform people into monsters. He says he saw people arriving at the FPH with *shiny, doll-like faces, baby-faces*, conjuring up a child's fantasy world, care-free and serene. He does not however take crime into consideration, crime that would deface that fantasy world and twist those doll-like faces out of recognition. He's convinced it is the FPH with all its insistence on treatment that is transforming the inmates into monsters. "Maybe you've treated their character problems or their moods, ok. But this torment you see in their faces, the dark circles under their eyes, you've made them suffer, you've destroyed them". For Matteo the medication performs a physical transformation; he accepts that it can have a positive effect on character and morals, but it "plants the monster on your face", it puts "dark circles under your eyes", it "makes you suffer", it "destroys you". What power there is in these images!

Some years later, I noticed that my patients in the Rehab Center made similar comments, "Doctor, I can feel the holes in my vein, but I'm not contagious"; "On the ward they helped me to expel the virus that was in me"; "Doctor, I'm taking Clozapine, but please, please, give me an antibiotic!". I mention this, because these statements confirm that the mentally disturbed (and particularly those suffering from schizophrenic psychoses) perceive their illness as being *contagious* and so in their view Clozapine can do little to restore them to health, what they really need is an antibiotic. They see the illness as contagious but there is an upside to this, it can also be eliminated, expelled (there's hope?).

Another interesting case is that of a patient being treated with Valproic acid and Clozapine (Leponex): "Leponex gives me hallucinations, I see things that aren't there, points of light, I hear ringing in my ears. I love dancing, but you need to have a clear head to dance. The *Leponex mask* makes me speak too quickly, makes me mad, do strange things". In another interview, he complained that "Clozapine gives me hallucinations, makes me bipolar. I dream of women dripping in blood. It's a hypnotic. It cancels my thoughts, then I forget things and I swear. I see molecules, particles. I've beaten up my conscience". "I read on *Famiglia Cristiana* that they experiment Leponex on snakes. It makes me ill; it doesn't cure me. It's hypnotic and I'm against hypnosis. I just want to take Depakin, nothing else. The priest prescribed me Depakin. The nurse gave me Prozac and Doctor M. gave me Modalina (trifluoperazine): I got mad, rabid, and like a dog excessive cerebralism to treatment, with dogs' sensitivity I always get furious. Leponex gives me visual and auditory hallucinations, I see shadows, molecules. Doctor T gave it me: I burned his clinic down. I can't take the *mask of madness*. Leponex makes me ill, it doesn't cure me."

The following comments were made by another patient, with a long history of substance abuse and psychoses, who was also being treated with Leponex. "When you take Leponex, it puts a psychiatric mask on you, it acts through hypnosis, it's been tested on dogs." Another patient said, "The wrong treatment made a mess of my brain. Now I don't need anything at all." Yet another, who lives in a world of delusions, packed with spies, secret service agents and international conspiracies, said "Clozapine makes my knees turn to water, it broke my ankles". Another patient suffering from a psychosis that distorts his perception of his identity, confided that "they are giving me too much Clozapine, it presses my brain against my skull, it's pure agony: I can't breathe or open my eyes", a sensation almost of physical death.

It's interesting to observe that this mechanism whereby the symptom is transferred from being the element that requires treatment to being a collateral effect of the treatment itself is also to be found in patients with neurosis. A young person who had never taken antipsychotics, but who had come to the Center asking for treatment for excessive outbursts of anger declared, "In general the idea of taking medicine for lunatics, antipsychotics, scares me. Just going to a psychologist makes me feel abnormal. Then my girlfriend took a course of anti-depressants and I saw her like, *crazy. Out of control.* If I take antipsychotics is there a risk you might lobotomize me?". This indicates that the phenomena of anxiety generated by a new prescription, an antipsychotic, and the attribution of collateral effects to the treatment that are in fact the symptoms of the illness itself, are to be found in cases of both psychosis and neurosis. It could then be hypothesized that this phenomenon is not produced by the cognitive sphere or consciousness, which remain intact in neurosis, but by the affective sphere which can be compromised in both neurotic and psychotic syndromes.

To recap, patients suffering from mental illnesses, schizophrenia in particular, tend to be wary of pharmaceutical treatments. In their view, the treatment causes their illness rather than curing it; the therapy creates a mask that distorts their real self. This is a phenomenon that we should be investigating; why does this happen in the treatment of mental illnesses, while it does not seem to occur in other specializations?

The number of collateral effects of antipsychotic drugs are legion: tardive dyskinesia, parkinsonism, the lowering of the epileptic threshold, emotional blunting, hypersalivation, increase in weight, fine tremors, lethargy, prolongation of the QT interval with a risk of arrythmia, possible alteration of the lipidic profile and the transaminases, possible long term negative effects on the thyroid and the liver, leukopenia, mood swings…

The patient who reads the leaflet tucked into the box of pills they have been prescribed will almost certainly take fright. It is up to the psychiatrist to explain how they work, the importance of taking them regularly and in the correct dosage and then to ensure that the instructions are followed to the letter. Regular blood tests should also be done where possible.

The use of multiple drugs may also contribute to this fear of pharmacological treatment. Sometimes patients in residential facilities (but also those who attend clinics) may be prescribed an additional therapy to respond to a particular symptomatology, without any adjustment being made to their original treatment. This may result in them taking a number of overlapping antidepressants and antipsychotic drugs with a heightened risk of incurring the collateral effects listed above, in particular tardive dyskinesia, parkinsonism, emotional blunting, hypersalivation, mood swings.

It is important therefore that the psychiatrist be precise when prescribing drugs. There is an extensive arsenal of products that can be used to attenuate symptoms such as delusions, paranoia, megalomania, jealousy, pervasive and persistent obsessions, manic and depressive crises, impulsive acts, acts driven by anger, explosive and uncontrollable bursts of anger against others and against oneself. Used appropriately, while maintaining a dialogue with the patient where possible, these products can achieve positive results.

The treatment, whether it be dialogue or anti-psychotics or a combination of both, must of course aim at attenuating the symptoms, or at least at helping the patient to accept and live with their symptom, or as Lacan said, their *sinthome,*[30] to the extent of *creating something new and enjoyable.* It should reduce, if not completely eliminate, the symptom of delusional disorder, so that the patient can live with it; moods should stabilize, there should be a decrease in the obsessive aspects, in the outbursts of anger and impulsiveness, thus preventing the occurrence of upsets.

As well as studying their patients' symptomatology and clinical history, the psychiatrist should listen carefully to their fears and concerns regarding the pharmacological treatment and, once the appropriate drug has been identified balancing its positive effects against the possible negative collateral repercussions, take responsibility for the treatment, regularly monitoring the evolution of the patients' state.

Luigi: That Old Man...

I Confessed to My Crime

During the show yesterday evening we talked about the FPHs closing down. They won't close by 2015. I read the papers and I know all about the extensions.

I am not worried about this little hiccup because in Catania, where I live, there are six rehab communities. I won't have any difficulty in getting accepted in one or another. This morning I got some good news from the priest here. I get on very well with him, I often go to see him.

---

[30] Lacan, J. (2016). *The Sinthome: The Seminar of Jacques Lacan, Book XXIII*. Polity Books. p. 106. ISBN 978-1-5095-1000-9.

I've got fifteen days leave now, and I'm going to stay with him. In December they'll review me being a danger to society and my lawyer has said that it will probably be dropped and I'll be a free man.

I'm here because I confessed to a murder that I committed. Because I had to bring up something that happened in 1986, or at least, that was when it started. I was only seven years old at the time; we were on the kerb in front of the villa, the "giardinetti" as they say in Lombardy, when I saw a man whose leg had been amputated. I pointed him out to my mother, saying, "Mamma, look, that man is just like my grandfather". But my grandfather had both legs. This man spat at my mother, called her a whore, and told her to teach her children manners. After that, things changed at home. Instead of coming home at seven o'clock, my father would stay out until two in the morning, he always took his meals alone and when he came home on Sundays, he would pull the tablecloth off the table and break all the plates. He always bought good plates from Tognana, not your common or garden plates. Once he even tore up his driving license. This was the atmosphere I grew up in, frightening and disruptive it was, so when I came across that old man again, I just wanted to kill him with my own hands. I said we beat him to death but actually he died of a heart attack. I said that because I wanted to vindicate my mother's honor. I gave myself up voluntarily, together with my brother and my cousin's boyfriend. We got sent down for twelve years and eight months. They changed my position with article 148[31] and I finished serving the sentence on November 22, 2008. I had three years on probation, but they reduced it to eighteen months. When my brother died, I cried in the rehab centre; there were some boys there that laughed at me, so I beat the daylights out of them with martial arts. I'm a ju-jitsu instructor; I did ju-jitsu from when I was thirteen to when I was nineteen.

I did my military service as an auxiliary with the carabinieri. I was a parachutist in Rome, I did some jumps and that's where I got this scar. I got a sprain, I let go the ripcord, the wind caught me and I hit a tree. I've explained the reason for my action, but it isn't justifiable for the purpose of saying "I'm in a lunatic asylum for a crime that would have been acceptable for prison".

[31] Art. 148 of the Italian penal code establishes that if a person is convicted of a crime then succumbs to a mental illness, they can be transferred to an FPH or similar institution.

Will They See My Story in the United States?

There's something vile in this. I have to say this. The vile part is that I involved my brother and got him arrested to protect him from protective custody. I did this for my cousin's boyfriend too. I said, "they didn't have anything to do with the murder, I did it alone." This is true, I did it alone. That man died of a heart attack, but I made that statement and stuck to it. They believed it because he had bruises around his right lung, I don't know how he got them. It was written on the post-mortem report. Maybe he got them when we turned him over, because we pinned him down on the bed with his hands behind his back, trussed him up like a goat. His heart gave out. It'll have been the shock of seeing three masked men jumping out on him and yelling, "You remember me? You offended my mother!", it would have scared the wits out of him. That'll be why he died. When we left him he was still alive. This doesn't mean that I'm trying to justify what we did and say that we shouldn't have gone to prison. I'm OK with that. At the end my mother and father made it up and now the family is happy again. That's good. I know, it's hard on me, that's what I'm saying. However in the end… I've got it. If my father had done that in 1986, instead of me doing it in 1999, I wouldn't be here. I wouldn't have had to cut myself because in prison were astonished I'd had my brother arrested. I didn't deny it and I never will. Why did I do it? To save him from protective custody. So one goes and not three. It was better that just one of us went into protective custody, because I'd killed an old man and that is a heinous crime. I didn't want all three of us to go because in protective custody you can't work, you can't study, you've got no rights at all. I know all about prison, I've done fifty-three months, thirty-four in high security regime for an old story, and now I'm here. I've been here from May 6, 2004, to November 22, 2008, then from December 7, 2010, till now. I did twenty-five months outside in a rehab community then they brought me back here when I beat up those people.

I want this interview to be transmitted on the Lombardy, Piedmont and Sicilian television news bulletins. Get it aired. Will they see it in the US? Because I've got relatives there. I want people to know that I'm not a monster that killed an old man for money, I killed him because my mother's honor was at stake. That's why I killed him. Because it just isn't worth going to prison for twelve years for seven million lire divided among three. My mother is very important to me. And more so now that she's no more. She's alive in heaven and in my heart so my mother is always with me. She protects me from above. I have a special angel who prays for me. That's a strong statement, but the truth must be told.

Virginio: An Error of Justice

I Studied Physics and Engineering. Then…

I was born in Taranto, I grew up in Rome, but I did high school in Taranto. I've been to several universities, Ferrara, Bologna, Turin. I studied Physics and Engineering.

When I was in high school my mother lived in Rome. My brother and sister had me sectioned when I came and we disagreed. The Involuntary commitment procedure is substantially illegal. It should be a guarantee because there are two doctors involved: one who proposes the procedure and the other who validates it, and there has to be a good reason for an involuntary commitment to the psychiatric ward of a hospital for seven days, renewable. But it is illegitimate because this procedure is applied too often. All that is needed is police intervention, two doctors' signatures and the mayor can't do anything about it, so this limitation of personal freedom and imposition of psychiatric treatment occurs quite frequently.

The FPH is substantially a procedure in which a judge comes up with a crime, he produces the crime as a pretext, all that is needed is a complaint, a police report with a medical report sent to a public prosecutor and he will order the confinement. This creates a vicious circle that is impossible to get out of. A guy who has a problem in the rehab community can be sent to a judge who will send him to the FPH. He'll send him there without a second thought and there he'll have to stay until who knows when. If you are accused of a crime, you can be imprisoned.

Anything can be a crime. I was on my way to the supermarket; it was ten to one and I was walking along a street off the beaten track. I was approached by a car, with two youngsters inside. They threatened me.

Then they backed up and came back from another direction. I kept on going towards the supermarket. There was a recycling bin there for bottles. The police accused me of smashing some bottles on the ground, of threatening some people (unknown), and to have damaged the door of a car that didn't stop. I went to the supermarket and did my shopping. When I came out, the police were waiting for me and they took me down to the station. They tried to do an involuntary commitment, but the psychiatrist said they couldn't because there were no grounds. The next day the police got a written report from the psychiatrist.

At that time, I was domiciled in the province of Turin, where I lived till I was confined. That was from 2008 to 2009, fourteen months all in Piedmont. They even accused me of touching a girl's bottom in 2003, imagine! I've been here since 2010, three years and four months. I've got reports that say I don't need to be in an FPH, and that I can be transferred to another service.

They took that report to the procurator, and they asked for imprisonment. I arrived here on June 2,[32] on a public holiday, as if it were a major operation. I've never set a foot outside since. They refuse to do anything for me because I was fit for trial, then I appealed, then I appealed to the Court of Cassation. And yet they could have looked for another place for me from the beginning. The FPH has never looked for another solution for me.

In October 1999 I was sectioned for seventeen days in the province of Brindisi. At the end of this involuntary commitment they gave me an injection. I went home. A few days later I started shaking, I was paralyzed, I couldn't get up from my bed. After three days they came and they said, "Virginio, shall we go the whole hog?" I said yes, and they did. I went into a coma. I stayed in a coma for several days, then there was the rehabilitation, I had catarrh in my lungs, they did a tracheotomy. I had bed sores too. When I fell out of bed the flesh died. They cut it away. They took my flesh away. They're not treating me here.

In my opinion the FPH was an error of judgement. I say it's impossible to unite the penal and the psychiatric. If you commit a crime, it's right that you go to prison, if on the other hand you commit a crime but it is

[32] June 2 is a national holiday in Italy, Republic Day.

obvious that your actions are caused by a psychic disorder, it's obvious you can't be imprisoned during that period.

I'm forty-eight years old. The FPH isn't a hospital or a clinic. OK, you have a problem for three days, you're not well, but surely that doesn't justify an involuntary commitment that lasts for years? With antipsychotics that destroy your personality and deny your dignity when there's a law that says that the maximum duration of an involuntary commitment is seven days. They already abuse it. The law is more protective. I didn't commit any crime. All I did was go to the supermarket and the police only said they saw broken bottles on the ground.

I'm Not a Psychiatric Specimen

There are people here who are aggressive, irrational, with a below average IQ, some are mute and there's no way of talking to them. What does mental illness mean? First, there is the concept of normality. Above all, you shouldn't be judged in a cage, together with others who have all kinds of problems and that become exacerbated in confinement. It's like an atomic reaction. It's impossible to judge a person on these grounds.

In my opinion I'm not suffering from any mental illness. I also think that the psychiatric reports don't say everything; they should put an end to that and tell the truth. There is no evidence of a psychiatric pathology. Let's not forget that lots of people have physical handicaps, they are physically deformed, and their faces are very different to what you expect to see in a person.

I hope that no one intends to break the law, the law that says these places have to close. The deadline was March 31, 2013. I was in Turin for a hearing, but they told me some people left, but then everything was blocked.

I'm in great difficulty because I was forty-five when I came here and I'm forty-eight now. I didn't have any problems and now I ask myself, what can I do to get a job in the outside world? My invalidity pension has been suspended, my apartment in Piedmont was devastated during my confinement; they'll have impounded it because it isn't worth much and the building expenses are high. My mother and brother, who live in Rome, emptied the place I had in Taranto. My mother lives in Rome, the apartment isn't hers, it belongs to my sister who bought it with my brother's help. My sister would like to live there with her husband and her son. My brother lives in EUR, he's an IT engineer, he's married with a son too and he has no intention of putting me up. So, what am I to do? I've got no future. A community? But I'm not a psychiatric specimen! My problem is to get out of here and have a role in society.

Francesco: I Turned on My Father

The Medication Ruined Me

I did eight months in prison then I came here. I've been here for three years and four months. One evening I fell out with my father. I've taken drugs. I took them in the 1990s then I stopped for ten years and opened a business. It was a sort of social club, some people that did cocaine came and one thing led to another, I took it up again myself. I went completely off the rails, I lost my job, I lost everything. I went to the Mental Health Service and they put me on Zyprexa, but that didn't do anything for me. They said it was a stimulator of … what did they say it was? Ah yes, an anti-psychotic, an equilibrator, a stabilizer, but it didn't do anything for me. I slept more. I took it in the morning and the evening, morning and evening, till one night I couldn't take it anymore, I exploded and started taking it out on my father for no reason. I even stabbed him; I pricked him on the stomach with the blade of a knife. Then in time I made peace with myself. I asked myself what the heck had I done? After working all those years then to go back and make the same mistake again? Now, I don't say I found an explanation but at least I found the motivation for the future. And to get out of this situation. So here I am, in this place. I feel much better. I've completely changed the medication. I feel better, much lighter. In a few days I'll go back to my town, to a Community there and I'll finish my sentence. I'll start working again and I'll recuperate all the good I did. This is the last sacrifice then I'll start working again. I've done a year here, and two in another FPH. I f**cked up, that's what. I'm almost fifty, I'm from Bari and I don't think I'll make the same mistake again.

People Fight Over a Cigarette

The FPH is useful but there isn't much control, there's not any real control over us patients; people that were fine, but lose it in here, people who aren't understood from the social standpoint. No, that's not right... from the human standpoint. If I end up in here, or people like me, we can manage; but folk who are weak, they die here, they end up getting seriously sick in here. And once they're sick there's no getting better, not in here or in a Community or anywhere else, because they're not self-sufficient because by then they're insane. And if you don't give these people a hand, they upset the others. You end up here because you've committed a crime, brawling, murder, drugs. A psychiatric illness means you don't have any control over yourself. That is, you commit a crime against a normal person without any motive. It's in the head, it's not a motivated thing.

Without a motive the matter isn't motivated, it's mental. Putting a person like that inside is right but you've got to keep an eye on them because if on the outside they got into a fight with a normal person, just imagine what they'll do in here where they fight over cigarette stubs. Most of the fights here are for cigarettes. Someone smokes a cigarette and throws the stub on the ground, the person behind him sees it—he doesn't have a cent to his name, poor soul, even his family has left him alone—goes and picks it up and smokes the filter. There's a guy who sees another guy smoking and goes and asks him for a cigarette and the other answers, "Get the hell outta here, or I'll kick your ass". A lot of people get into real fights this way.

Being a danger to society makes you understand that you are still being assessed and that you still aren't normal. According to them, you're dangerous. When they decided I was a danger to society I was in a state of confusion. I was in prison and they ... I'm here but I should be in prison, but they did that psychiatric thing, what do you call it? Yes, that's it, a psychiatric assessment. And they said that thing there: unfit to plead. That's it: unfit to plead. I wasn't able to plead. That was Greek to me. I'd never heard of it before. They sent me here. Danger to society, unfit to plead, these are things I discovered here. The guys who know their way around here, they explained it all to me. I'm not a danger to society, not at all. I only did it once in my life, that time with my father, I'd never been in a fight before. I got caught up in drugs in the 80s; my friends dragged me into that mess because I'd never have been able to do it on my own. So I got into a mess… then I stopped. In 2000 I started again, then I stopped; I didn't touch the stuff again for years.

Then for a crappy incident, I can't relapse for a crappy thing like that, again. That's it. I've done everything else, so I had to do time and then the FPH. I've learnt a lot though. I'm tougher now. I'm someone to be reckoned with. Oh yes, because when you are in here you miss your freedom, you really understand what it means to be free. You really appreciate it. Here you have time, from morning to night, to think about your past. Here you have all the time in the world. You think over what you've done in your life, in society and you weigh it all up. I've always worked, that's one good thing I've done. I never went to school; I started working when I was very young. I've always worked. Here they let me take the middle school diploma, then I got another three, a diploma for working in the library, one for hygiene and cleanliness, and one for attending cooking courses.

Work is everything, it is life itself, it is bread, peace. It's how you take your own measure, it helps you to grow, you have to grow with ideals, become mature, then the experiences that you have you transmit to others. I've helped others. Work is a lot of things to me. As soon as I get out of here I'll find a job, have a family, because when I was taking drugs I lost everything: my fiancée, my friends… Now I'm a bit at loggerheads with my father but things are working out. Oh yes, fighting with your father after years and years of him bringing you up, of living together. And you have to go and have a fight with your father! Well, he's a bit surly, a bit on the hard side… he's one of the old school, my father. There are four of us in my family. My brothers talk a bit about what I'm doing here, so now, after never wanting to hear my name mentioned again, every so often he talks about me: that's better than nothing.

They came up from Bari and they were impressed by how well I am, and they'll come and get me in a month's time. I'll get my medication changed. At the moment, I don't see any difference between when I take it and when I don't. Actually Zyprexa ruined me. It just ruined me. Between the medication and the drugs, I just couldn't take any more. I exploded.

I Found My Faith in the FPH

Here in the FPH I got close to the Church. I've found faith here. Three years ago I heard that you can go to mass on Sundays and I went. I used to go as a kid. I went one Sunday; it's not a big church, holds just a hundred or so people. I liked it. Then there was Padre Pippo, he came in the mornings from 9.30 to 11.30 and I've never left him since and I'll never leave the Church again. I've read the New Testament; I've bought a Bible. I want to read it all. It helps me morally. There are some parts in it that tell about things that happened then, that have happened to me now. I'm here, I've done nothing other than learn to understand what I did, learn what I have to do when I get out. It's a passage between one reality and another. I've learned this maturity here. If you don't experience things yourself, you can't understand them. If I tell the doctor my head feels strange, he'll give me medication but he won't be able to understand what I'm feeling. If you haven't experienced it, you can't understand what you feel in your brain. It's not easy to explain.

Prison and FPH are restrictive places, there aren't enough controls. If they were better monitored… for example, in a place like this we spend the whole day doing nothing.

In the FPH, as long as you are following a cure it's OK, they keep an eye on you, but as soon as you're better, you're active. I've taken four diplomas, I'm active, why don't you find me a job on the outside? They brought me here and for eleven months I laid on my bed from morning till night. Why don't you find me a job on the outside? I could sleep here at night, then go to work in the morning and earn some money so I could buy myself a coffee, go to a restaurant. There's no sense to this FPH, it's got no basis, it's got nothing to teach anyone. It's not a clinic. It's huge. They say it's the biggest in Europe. All the staff in administration, the guards, doctors, educators, they could do so much more. They put your name on a list for courses. Who cares about doing a course? They leave you there from morning till night. They don't take you anywhere, they don't help you, they leave you on your bed from morning till night, you stay on your bed, someone cleans the room, you go for a walk and so on. The brain, you know… come today, come tomorrow… the day after tomorrow. Then you call home: have you spoken to the lawyer? What did he say? He says that you'll be out soon. Lies. Just empty lies. There are lots of rumours here. If you aren't strong psychologically, you freak out. I've seen lots end up that way. I've seen perfectly normal people turning into lunatics after a while; they accused Christ, they yelled, got into fight after fight, lit up their rooms, smashed up sinks, baths, beds, they cut themselves. When I saw all this happening, I said to myself, where on earth have they put me?

What did they diagnose me with? I don't know, they didn't let me read it. I was confused at the time, I remember that during the assessment they showed me photos, they asked me questions, there was no reason that I should have fought with my father like that. It was the drugs. What illness do I have? What symptoms? I've no idea. No, I don't know.

In the FPH I've kept myself busy, otherwise I'd never leave the room. I attended the school. Every day there was a different teacher. We were in groups, in the morning. It was nice. In the afternoon, it was a dormitory, a cemetery. You went to the infirmary because you had a headache and asked for something to take for it. "Can't you come back later?", would be the response. But my head hurts now! Maybe it was better when there was a fight, at least it brightened up the atmosphere a bit. Incredible.

Therapy: Drugs

Then I had therapies. A bit of everything. I went all over Puglia looking for a doctor who knew his stuff and could tell me why it wasn't the drugs that made me unwell, it was the pill, a drug in the form of a pill. I bought them in the chemist, and they were drugs, with a cocaine base, amphetamines. I went there with my prescription, I gave them my documents, I gave them seven thousand lire and they gave me a little bottle. I felt great and I could go for three days without eating and sleeping, I was fine, sharp, strong, always working. Then everything crashed, everything, my head too, after seven months. So they told me to give over taking that medicine and go on to heroin and cocaine instead. I wasn't with it. And I said to them, "What have you made me take?" and they said "Don't you worry, we got our heads together with this. Go on, try it, try it!" and I tried it, like a cretin. In those days, in the 1980s, there wasn't the information that there is today, it was all underground. So there I was, in that period, trying everything, hidden away. Dreams. We were just kids. Today we know everything, the illnesses the drugs cause, the harm they do. I heard them talking on television about the new drugs… the youngsters will ruin themselves… They are kids. I fell for it… but after I was twenty. These days they are just kids. What a life.

What are my expectations? I want to have a family because I didn't before, I want a job, get a driving licence and try to sort things out with my mother and father. No more fighting. A regular lifestyle, healthy, humble, law-abiding. Go to Church. Woe betides me if I don't … this is a hobbyhorse of mine. Live an orderly life. I did before, but it was disorderly. You know, without the Church. I opened shop when I felt like it, after all I was the owner. Sometimes I opened, sometimes I didn't, there was always enough money, it was a good life. But these were the things that got me off the rails. These days I keep my eyes open. I don't need drugs anymore. They're not good for anything, they just muck your head up, and you don't understand anything anymore. While you're taking them you feel fine, I know because I've been there. I felt great, but then you pay the consequences twice over. You pay the price of the drugs when you're high, but then you pay it again when you're normal, like I am now. I'm not like that now, I'm down, I'm crushed under my own weight, I can't breathe anymore, I can't lift my head up. Doing drugs is bad, bad, bad, bad. If you aren't strong you fall into depression, I've seen others fall into depression, they told me all about it and said that they saw everything black, and when someone tells you they see everything black you know they have lost the desire to live, to go ahead. There's no continuation, no life, breath, friendship, peace: there are none of these things anymore. It's dangerous. Much better to give it up.

5

The Forensic Psychiatric Hospital of Montelupo Fiorentino

The Forensic Psychiatric Hospital of Montelupo Fiorentino

Ten years after the first FPH in Italy was opened in Aversa, the second was opened in Montelupo Fiorentino; it was housed in the seventeenth century Villa Medicea, known locally as the Ambrogiana, and had already had a chequered history. It was the summer residence of Ferdinando I de' Medici, Grand Duke of Tuscany. He had purchased the land in 1574 and restructured the existing buildings, transforming them into an imposing square edifice with four square corner towers on the angles. In the second half of the seventeenth century, Cosimo III de' Medici adopted it as his official residence, and the villa prospered. A devout man, he had a convent built there for the Friars Minor from Spain and a church dedicated to Saints Lucia, Quirico, and Pietro d'Alcantra. In the nineteenth century, under Leopold II, the last reigning grand duke of Tuscany, the villa fell on hard times. It was practically abandoned and the construction of the first Italian railroad, known as the Leopolda, which traversed the approach road to the villa, cutting it off from the town, convinced Leopold II, the last reigning Grand Duke of Tuscany, to use it for social

J. Santambrogio, *Stories from Italian Forensic Psychiatric Hospitals*,
https://doi.org/10.1007/978-3-031-61129-2_5

purposes. The initial project, to transform the villa into a lunatic asylum, was abandoned as being too costly and it was used as a prison instead, with male prisoners being housed in the villa itself and female prisoners in the convent. Thirty years later, in 1886, it became a criminal asylum.[1]

The transformation of the villa in Montelupo Fiorentino into a criminal asylum was dictated by necessity as in the wake of the unification of Italy in 1861, Aversa was the only confinement structure in Italy to have a section for the criminally insane. The task of transforming the Ambrogiana into an institution suitable to accommodate the overflow from Aversa was entrusted to a man who had made a name for himself in this sphere of activity. Dr. Leopoldo Ponticelli was the director of the agricultural penal colony on the island of Pianosa and during his tenure had greatly improved the buildings and the condition of the inmates. He introduced work in the fields, researched the crops that could be grown on the island and enhanced the agronomic techniques in collaboration with experts of the sector. Pianosa became a model institution; the vineyards flourished, wine was produced and flowers were cultivated. Ponticelli insisted on having qualified personnel working on the island, capable of treating possible medical emergencies arising from the island environment. When the director general of prisons, Martino Beltrami Scalia, asked Ponticelli to identify a suitable location for another criminal asylum, he chose Montelupo Fiorentino as being in a central position and easily reached by rail, the same railway that had been seen as a drawback by Leopold II. Ponticelli took on the task of supervising the restructuring of the building and used the prisoners already confined there for manpower, significantly reducing the cost of the project. In 1886 the final transformation phase was completed; the Ambrogiana was fitted out with the medical and scientific equipment for its new role, and appropriate clothes were ordered for the patients. Ponticelli even obtained a special van to transport the *lunatics* from the railway station to the criminal asylum. He was nominated first director of Montelupo Fiorentino.

---

[1] Conti, P. (2016). L'OPG di Montelupo Fiorentino. In Grassi, G., Bombardieri, C. (eds.) *Il Policlinico della Delinquenza. Storia degli Ospedali Psichiatrici Giudiziari italiani*. Franco Angeli.171–182.

The Ambrogiana was to accommodate several infamous inmates including Giovanni Passannante, the anarchist who attempted to assassinate King Umberto I in 1878. He died there in 1910. Another would-be assassin of the king, Pietro Acciarito, was imprisoned there from 1897 until his death in 1943. Cesare Lombroso, the founder of criminal anthropology, wrote a paper on anarchists, expounding the anarchic personality.[2] He was convinced that "all those accused of strange or atrocious crimes, crimes without an apparent motive or crimes where the motive is out of proportion compared to the crime itself" should be confined in criminal asylums.[3]

A full history of the Ambrogiana has never been written and unfortunately the documentation regarding the patients confined in the institution from 1886 to 1950 has been badly damaged by damp. However, at least two documents are available. The first is a report written by a Milanese law professor, Raffaele Nulli, at the end of the criminal asylum's first year of operation; it was published in 1887 under the title *Una visita al nuovo Manicomio Criminale dell'Ambrogiana e l'istituzione dei Manicomi Criminali in Italia* (A Visit to the new Ambrogiana Criminal Asylum and the institution of Criminal Asylums in Italy).[4] Professor Nulli visited the Ambrogiana accompanied by Dr. Ponticelli and the resident psychiatrist Dr. Algeri; his report is considered by scholars to be culturally important and part of the knowledge base of civilization and as such has been conserved and reprinted. At that time the structure had capacity for 208 prisoners and 52 persons waiting for sentencing; the inmates were 97, with 18 prison guards and 11 nurses. The second document is a graduation thesis written in 1988 by Paola Paoli;[5] she extrapolated as much data as possible from the files of the first ten years of operation and was able to compile a report. She noted that the number of inmates arriving from

[2] Lombroso, C. (1895). *Gli Anarchici.* Fratelli Bocca.

[3] Lombroso, C. (1872). Sull'Istituzione dei Manicomi Criminali in Italia. In *Rendiconti al Regio Istituto di Scienze, Lettere ed Arti.* Turin.

[4] Nulli, R. (1887). *Una Visita al Nuovo Manicomio Criminale dell'Ambrogiana e l'Istituzione dei Manicomi Criminali in Italia* (Classic Reprint)(Italian Edition). Forgotten Books. ISBN 978-1332387205.

[5] Paoli, P. (Academic Year 1989–1990). *Il Manicomio Criminale dell'Ambrogiana alla fine dell'Ottocento. Contributi allo studio di una istituzione totale.* Doctoral thesis conserved in the Library of Montelupo Fiorentino.

prisons increased over time to 140; the majority were young (over 50% were less than 34 years of age), 90 came from the south of Italy and of the remaining 50, 25 came from north Italy and 25 from central Italy. Of the patients coming from the north, 20% were from Cuneo and 16% from Turin; of those coming from the central region, 24% came from Rome and 20% from Perugia, while from the south and islands, 10% came from Agrigento, 8% from Bari and 7.7% from Caltanissetta and from Sassari. 127 had no economic means, 2 owned a small piece of land, 8 were landowners, 1 was wealthy, 1 was well off and 1 for whom no information was registered; 69 were farmers (or farm workers), 28 craftsmen, 39 laborers, and 4 with no information given. The majority of the farm workers came from the south, while most of the laborers and craftsmen were from the north, which reflected the situation in the country, where the north was becoming increasingly industrialized while the south remained prevalently rural. Most of the patients were single (66.4%) and had no children (76.4%). The thesis also records the patients' state of health, providing an interesting, though somewhat imprecise classification as the institution did not provide clear information regarding the mental and physical health of the inmates. So, 47 (33.6%) were declared to be "mad, chronically mad, weird, manic with hallucinations", 23 (16.4%) were considered to be "epileptic, vain, idiotic, and lethargic", 59 were described as "good, bad, mediocre, fair, bathetic". No comments were registered for 11 patients. Regarding the level of education, 64 (45.7%) were illiterate, 52 (37.2%) were able to read and write, 3 were only able to sign their name and no information was given for 21 inmates. In 125 (89.3%) cases, the reason for confinement was given as crimes against persons, 14 were guilty of crimes against property and in 1 case the crime was not recorded. Although work was known to be therapeutic, only 4 inmates actually worked; the remaining 136 (97.1%) were unemployed. Of the 4 who did have employment, 2 worked in the garden, one was a bricklayer and one did repairs. Ms Paoli drew the following conclusions: "The majority of the inmates who left the Criminal Asylum alive were transferred to the Civil Asylum because although they had settled their debt with the law, they were still suffering from the mental illness that had afflicted them when they entered the Criminal Asylum. Only in a very limited number of cases, where the illness was less severe, was the inmate restored to his family and remained under their surveillance. Finally, there were many cases of prisoners from prisons, penal colonies and similar institutions of detention, which supports the theory that considers the prison system generated madness."[6]

In 1986, one hundred years after the opening of the Ambrogiana, Dr. Franco Scarpa became the director of the institution, which in the meantime had become an FPH. He wrote: "When I took on the position of director, Montelupo Fiorentino was rather unique as it was hampered by a difficult relationship with the surrounding territory. I arrived just when a memorandum of understanding was being signed by Dr. Amato, my predecessor, that would lead to the closing of the FPH. This, on the one hand. On the other, I found very good relationships with the outside. The institution had just been through a period in which it had been heavily penalized by the presence of a number of inmates who were members of criminal organizations. This meant that the FPH had to be closely monitored and cut off from the outside, with tough security measures. The situation is gradually normalizing, relations with the external environment are being restored and additional health services are being taken on."[7]

Seventeen years later, he described the situation in the Ambrogiana as follows: "Today we have about 190 inmates, most of whom come from the center-north, very few from Sicily, Campania and Puglia. The average age is 40 years, and the average length of confinement, keeping in mind we have security measures of 2, 5 and 10 years, does not exceed four to four and a half years. This means we have very few inmates who have been here for over 10 years. While up to 1984 the inmates of the FPH were prevalently connected to organized crime, today the patients are genuinely suffering from mental illnesses and to a certain extent this is due to a failure in today's society. I'm talking here about young psychotics, people who commit crimes in the family, where social relations are increasingly acute. The level of education is very low. But the situation is slowly changing. We are starting to see very young boys with diplomas

---

[6] Paoli, P. (Academic Year 1989–1990). *Il Manicomio Criminale dell'Ambrogiana alla fine dell'Ottocento. Contributi allo studio di una istituzione totale.* Doctoral thesis conserved in the Library of Montelupo Fiorentino.

[7] Inchiesta sull'OPG di Montelupo Fiorentino. Incontro con Franco Scarpa. http://www.ristretti.it/areestudio/salute/mentale/citta/montelupo.htm.

from high school who have committed crimes. Only 50% of the inmates have accepted employment, unfortunately. The main problem with psychiatric patients is how to stimulate them. I want to emphasize here that work is important. It is a fundamental, constructive step in the path to rehabilitation, helping the inmate to find employment in a social cooperative, or some other form of work locally. We start with an orientation course run by an expert in job placement that covers motivation, identifies typologies, experience and competences. Once this phase has been completed successfully, an apprenticeship is found with a social cooperative or a local company and, finally, a full-scale job."[8]

Franco Scarpa was the chief medical officer of the FPH Montelupo Fiorentino until 2015. In 2008 he handed over the administrative aspects to Dr. Antonella Tuoni.

I visited Montelupo Fiorentino at the end of 2014, just months before the last inmate left in February 2015. It was a period of transformation and I had many questions, which in the course of time were to find answers. At the end of my visit, I met with Dr. Franco Scarpa and had the opportunity of discussing my experiences with his collaborators, Maria Rosaria Capone and Luca Bigalle (psychiatrists), and Antonella Lettieri (psychologist). During these meetings I was impressed by their professional dedication, their vision of the illnesses and the treatments, their interest in the individual patients as human beings. A summary of the conversations I had with these professionals is given here; they reflect the painstaking work undertaken in a complex and controversial institution and above all, the motivation behind their passion for caring for these patients with their unexpectedly fragility.

Interview with the Director, Franco Scarpa

Let me introduce myself. I am a doctor, specializing in neurology, criminology, and psychiatry. I started my career in Aversa, as deputy chief medical officer. I spent a year and a half there, then of my own volition I transferred to Montelupo Fiorentino as chief medical officer. It was 1986.

[8] Inchiesta sull'OPG di Montelupo Fiorentino. Incontro con Franco Scarpa. http://www.ristretti.it/areestudio/salute/mentale/citta/montelupo.htm.

Working in a FPH was a formidable challenge for me, as it was for all health workers, every day you have to face a reality characterized by two decidedly contrasting aspects: mental illnesses and a violation of the law which in many cases was associated with violence, causing harm and pain to others. This meant that you had to treat the person, keeping in mind both their mental disorder and their violent behavior, all in the framework of a prison environment. These people were not in hospital of their own free will, and this had a negative impact on both the therapeutic relationship and the patients' inclination to follow the prescribed treatment. Our objective as doctors, therefore, was to treat the disorder but also to create the conditions in which it would be possible for the magistrate, who had the final decision as to the duration of the security measure, to evaluate the degree of social danger posed by the patient and, in those cases where this had been reduced or eliminated, revoke it.

The closure of the criminal psychiatric asylums was a positive step. This does not mean ignoring the existence of patients with difficult and complex issues who need particular attention and resources. Psychiatric pathologies are also affected by external events, crises, an imbalance in socio-environmental conditions, family situations that cannot be managed either by the family members or the local health services; they need specialized structures and step-by-step treatment, where sometimes the step must be backwards and not forwards to find the appropriate treatment to avoid a relapse. In my experience, there are many patients who are afflicted by pathologies that are not only psychiatric in nature. These patients suffer from more than one disorder, they have multiple complex pathologies, and many problems. They are assigned to psychiatric services, which are then obliged to deal with all types of problems. This puts psychiatry, in a position of weakness as it has to manage problems that involve a plethora of factors: organicity, drug and alcohol abuse, social situations that are even more difficult to treat in a psychiatric patient.

Patients or prisoners? When treating psychiatric disorders, we often forget to answer that fundamental, basic question: who are these people? One of my collaborators in the FPH once reported to me what one of the inmates had said to him and I will never forget it, "when I go into the infirmary I feel like a patient, as soon as I set foot in the corridor outside the infirmary I feel like a prisoner." I often ask myself, and how do we—doctors, nurses, health workers—how do *we* consider *them*? If their crime is upmost in our minds, then they are prisoners. But these are people, psychiatric patients and their crime must be seen within the framework of their history. I'm not a supporter of the concept of social danger. It should be rediscussed and rethought because it has become a chimera, a hybrid. Social danger with an expiry date. If fitness to stand trial is evaluated with an eye to the past, I mean taking into account the crime committed in that specific moment in time, social danger inevitably becomes a projection into the future and the evaluation is made considering what might happen in the future (article 203 of the Italian Penal Code). How can we predict when an earthquake will happen? In many countries the methods used to evaluate risk are more accurate: an evaluation is made of the risk of violence, transgressive actions, recidivism. Once the level of risk has been established, appropriate courses of treatment can be applied as well as monitoring activities and risk management programs.

Tests. In the judicial field, clinical judgement must always be supported by instruments for objective evaluation, particularly when dealing with social danger. In addition to the classic diagnostic scales such as SCID, MMPI and other such, I strongly recommend using tests like the HCR-20 (Historical, Clinical, Risk Assessment) which, in the recent version 3, accurately assesses the risk of violent behavior and the scenarios that profile such risks and programs for their management and control.

The psychiatric patient opens an important theme: ***rehabilitation***. But first, it is important to clarify what is meant by rehabilitation. It is the recuperation of independence, the capacity to exert civil rights, to be a citizen, to exert self-control. Psychiatric patients must be treated: they have the right to rehabilitation, and at the same time they must recover their rights. When they are treated and the psychiatrist works on what is undamaged in their being, they gradually manage to face their guilt. This is a gradual task that requires skill. In prison this task comes up against impediments; the punishment in no way touches the guilt.

I have always been against ***restraint***. When I arrived in Montelupo it was used frequently and one of the first things I did was to reduce the number of rooms in which it was carried out; finally there was only one room with two/three beds for restraint. Two thirds of the inmates who were subjected to this procedure were ex-prisoners and one of the main reasons was aggressivity. There were fewer of these cases when the cells were opened after the 1990s. Previously they were kept locked twenty-four hours a day. Only a few remained closed for complex cases and cases of risk. The possibility of being able to move outside the cell, normally occupied by five or six inmates, reduced the tensions that such proximity inevitably caused. We carried out a study on the decisions taken and the consequences, and it soon became clear that opening the cells reduced aggressivity but required work to keep the tone of discussions down and techniques to limit and avoid risk of escalation. As preventative measures we adopted a system of monitoring cell cohabitation and ensured the constant attention of psychiatrists to the study of the optimum combinations of patients in the cells.

Interview with Antonella Lettieri (Psychologist) and Maria Rosaria Capone (Psychiatrist)

In the FPH there has always been the need to take care of patients and their families experiencing their first contact with serious crime and confinement. These families are the most fragile. We conducted an experiment with a group of six families with sons who had committed murder when in a sudden state of psychotic imbalance. All were young men who were employed and had never shown any problematic behavior previously. These families needed to understand what had happened and why; they also needed information regarding the FPH, which was always perceived as a place where *monsters* are confined. They wanted to face up to the guilt, the shame, learn how to deal with it. The parents felt responsible, they told how they had shut themselves in their homes for six months, how frightened they felt and how they couldn't look people in the eye. One father told us that when finally he found the courage to leave his home, he only went out at a particular time of day, and walked close to the walls so as not to be noticed.

We held meetings in which the participants were helped to contextualize what had happened, and to face the murder and the sense of guilt. All of them felt strongly that they had failed their son, they had not read the situation correctly, they hadn't understood his distress, and had waited too long before contacting a doctor or the health services. Our role was to listen, provide support, and in part, psychotherapeutic assistance. We worked on the emotional aspects and the group started to respond and to express their grief, sharing it with the others. We believe that this is an important initial step, helping the families to make sense of the situation; they in turn help their sons to participate in their grief.

The project stimulated a sense of solidarity among the families who participated; they developed relationships and a form of self-help that we hope will not be lost. They even created an association *Families of patients in FPHs* which was active on the internet. The experiment continues although it is increasingly evident that these services require a project design, involvement, and resources. The closure of the FPH has raised a number of questions in this sense, particularly from the families who ask, "what will happen to us after the FPH closes? Will our son be treated properly, from a medical point of view? Where? Who will be our point of reference?". We believe that this experience could provide guidelines for the future rehabilitation centers.

Interview with Luca Bigalli (Psychiatrist)

Is it possible to treat patients in a FPH? This was the question that always tormented me in Montelupo, from the day I arrived in 1995. The FPHs, like prisons (where I've also worked), are characterized by segregation and suffering. This greatly influences and conditions the activities. But is it possible to treat patients there? Yes, just as in any other location, keeping in mind however certain conditions. The power of the therapy depends on the group, rather than on the institution. It can't be denied that the environment is important: overcrowding should be avoided, there should be adequate and appropriate spacing, such as keeping the cafeteria separate from the toilets (it may sound obvious, but in prisons this unfortunate coupling of service areas is frequently to be found). There is no respect of privacy. Over the years we have informed the authorities of malfunctions and repairs urgently required. Politicians, commissions, and other types of association have come to the FPH in Montelupo but nothing ever came of these visits. Not even when we ourselves asked them to return. They turned a deaf ear. Only the Commission led by Ignazio Marino produced a change. I welcome the closure of the FPHs. The transition to prevalently medical structures respects the dignity of the people involved, but it must guarantee what the prison structure did not offer. In my view the rehabilitation centers and the new treatment institutions must learn from the history and the limitations of the FPHs, and they must also take into consideration the problematics that we have had to face on a daily basis with all the relative dynamics. My experience, and the experiences of my colleagues, leads me to say that the FPHs reflected and responded to the contradictions of society; they satisfied a need. We received patients who hadn't been appropriately treated or who had not allowed anyone to treat them. These patients often came from the health services. It was really distressing when a patient we had treated, cured, and discharged, and who then should have been supported by external services, returned to the FPH. Too few rehabilitation centers, not enough qualified medical staff. A defeat for the region and a defeat for the FPH. These situations are an indication as to what happens outside, the complexity of the disorders and the need for planning.

If I were to evaluate my years in the FPH, I would say that despite the limitations and the conditions there were some great successes, in particular when patients started to come to terms with their disorders. Those who have committed serious crimes have only two options open: either they manage to overcome their disorder (helped by treatment) or they condemn themselves to a failed existence. When you manage to help a person to restore their plans for their future it is a success.

Dario: Rehabilitation

The Sea Lulled Me to Sleep

I've had lots of jobs. Got experience. Been a window dresser, dressed shop windows, I mean I set them up, and there were competitions for the best arrangements, where you had to arrange things in a particular way… I mean, I was an apprentice, that's often much better than studying, right?

I've good taste, I love life, know what I mean? *This isn't life, this place is a dump, a shithole… it's a shithole, get it?*

They got me for stalking. They accused me of stalking two girls. My ex who aborted my son when I was twenty-one. She aborted my son; he was a fetus, at three months he was as big as a six-month fetus, you know? She's accusing me of going to her house, said she had to move to another place… I never gave a flying f*ck for her, really, I don't even know where she lives. We lost touch for twenty-four years. Then there was this social worker who certainly… well, I got on her nerves… OK, I realize I made a balls-up there… but I don't deserve being in a place like this, get what I mean? I've got potential, mind and body potential. I can do anything, you know? I used to go windsurfing, bodysurfing, sailing a catamaran, laser, I competed in regattas. My old man worked in a club, I've sailed regattas with world champions, know what I mean? I love the sea, know what I mean? I'm a fisherman, I'm used to being lulled to sleep by the waves and wake up the same way. In the morning I'd lower my nets, a couple of kilometers of nets and I'd earn four-five hundred euros a day, you know? I earn good money when I work.

Difficulties in Adolescence

I'm here in this place. That's clear enough, isn't it? It pisses me off. I did time in Aversa too: I did four years in the Criminal Asylum there because I destroyed two cars that were parked in my two personal parking places: I mean, there was a notice saying "Private Property" right there in the parking place. I'd told them before they couldn't park there… and instead they parked there again with the same cars I'd found there before. In other words, they kept on using my private parking spaces, so I smashed their cars up with a baseball bat. Where I come from, if you don't show you've got guts, they wipe their shoes on you, know what I mean? Get the idea? A small town full of bullies, where the strongest dictates the law, where the families join forces?

Yep, I was in Aversa before. To be honest, I had some problems, not existential problems, but just a feeling of not fitting in right from when I was sixteen. You know, when you're neither fish nor fowl, you're a teenager and you can't figure out what you're doing here? I came into this world in a family that was always arguing about something… my brother-in-law comes in and my father starts yelling at him because my sister ought to have been home at a certain time… see… it was all a bit of a mess: my mother defending my sister, my father losing his temper with my mother. My old man died of cancer in 2000, you see… my life hasn't all been sweetness and light, not by a long chalk. What to say? I had a psychoanalyst at 16, not your psychologist or anything like that, eh. A psychoanalyst! Yes, she helped, she opened up my life a bit. She's alright: her name is Patrizia I don't know if she's from Cagliari or not, her surname doesn't sound as if she's from Cagliari, doesn't even sound Sardinian. I went to Cagliari, to the Civil Hospital. Symptoms? I felt distressed, *I had a problem*. When I went out, I felt awkward, you know, people… I asked questions that my parents couldn't answer, they just weren't able to. My psychoanalyst told me that certain things are normal; everyone asks certain questions. My parents were a little… let's say my father got to the third year in secondary school, my mother the third year in elementary school, get it? Like they weren't exactly cultured… I did third year in secondary school but I taught myself pedagogy, I helped my girlfriend do her final exams at high school.

I heard on television the other day that a maths teacher molested his pupils, he blackmailed them, wanted sex in exchange for passing them on exams. That's sick… I can't stand pedophiles. Now, my educator, she's fifty-two and I'm forty-seven. I'm no pedophile, f*ck it. She f*cked up morally and ethically, not me. Like, if you're an educator you can't get into bed with the person you're supposed to be educating. Like, I'm forty-seven, but I feel quite mature, got it?

No, Aversa really… ye gods… Aversa is bad, man… really bad. I was in the Staccata.[9] I was in ward 5, then in 8bis, that's where Cutolo[10] escaped from, where they blasted the wall down. I was in all the sections and then I was in a ward where there weren't any prison guards.

[9] The section reserved for criminals with long sentences and little hope of recovery.

[10] Raffaele Cutolo was a notorious Italian criminal who founded the Nuova Camorra Organizzata.

I F*cked Myself Up with an Educator

Then I went to a rehab center in Sardinia, Morgongiori, it's called, run by a priest. Not that the priest did much, all the work was done by ex-drug addicts. I worked there, took care of the animals, worked on the land, in the nursery garden—I planted lettuce, fennel, tomatoes, courgettes, aubergines, spinach, lots of stuff.

I've a lot of experience and so I don't feel like I should be here, know what I mean? I can't stay here, I just can't. I've got a good lawyer, who really has my interests at heart because she's my brother's girlfriend even if my brother's married to someone else…

I take Carbolithium, that's lithium salts. Salts that you get from fruit but I need more… no, it's not that I need more, it's that I don't assimilate them. So, I have to take them … but I don't take anything else, I take 150 mg in the morning and 150 mg in the evening. I've been in prison where people take buckets of medicine, you know? I could have gone to prison, easy like, rather than coming here. But my doctor… no, the deputy public prosecutor, instead of talking to me, he went and talked to this doctor, who I'm sure is protecting Signora Antonina, my ex-educator. They really humiliated me, you know?

This educator, she got interested in me. She came to my house, we ate together. I've got witnesses who saw us snogging, not actually doing it but it was clear that we were an item. I'm sorry about that. I don't hate her: I don't hate her because I understand that she was just trying to protect her kids, you know? She's got a boy of thirteen and one of fourteen, he's cool. I would never do anything to harm someone like her because she did a lot for me. I understand her. It was my psychiatrist who f*cked up there, you know? He talked to the deputy public prosecutor and, instead of talking to me to see if I could go to prison, they decided I should go to a Rehab Community. There, I had no one to talk to, no dialogue, because those people are really demented, mentally not with it. There were a couple who had come from the FPH and I was about to get into trouble with them, but I got out of it: I kept myself to myself most of the time. In fact, I called my lawyer and asked her to talk to the people in charge, instead of staying with us inmates they are always in the office, doing admin stuff. They never come to talk to us. There are very few educators… like there are educators and health care workers that deal with the people, OK? Being here is a real problem for me… it's very bad: not that it gets to me at all… I don't let anything get to me anymore. I survived Aversa, I survived the Staccata in Aversa … now, if you know what that is…. *mamma mia*… do you know the Staccata?

I Prefer Prison, Here They Yell Too Much

I wasn't in prison long enough, because then they sent me to the FPH. This really penalizes me. It makes me feel how I don't want to feel; I don't like feeling like this. Morally many times… just as well there are people here I know, like maybe even if you've done some really bad stuff it's OK with them. Lots of them are in a really bad way. There are people here who can't remember things from one day to another… I've never seen them write a letter, read, they're not like me, you know? It's different in prison: you've got a life, you can play football, the people there are the same as me, you can play cards… even if it sounds like no big deal… it's a totally different life, I feel I'm being really, really penalized here. Here in Montelupo I feel like I'm being held back, badly held back. Prison is much more constructive, much more constructive. I've asked them to find me a job, but I'm not working. I used to work, I worked for almost a year and I liked it. That's it. Here they yell from morning till night, there are people who are away with the fairies, get what I mean? And I've got to put up with this day and night. It's really bad for a person who is involved in… I don't know if you know Osho, the Indian guru? I did biological nutrition, so purity of body and soul is important to me, you know? I really don't like being here, I don't, I don't I don't. What really gets to me is that I've got a social life out there and that to get out of here I'll probably have to do time in another rehab. I'm forty-seven years old, I don't have any more time to waste, get what I mean?

I'm in the Pesa ward. I hope they don't move me up to Arno because I've seen it… and it's filthy, but really filthy… If they put me in Arno, I'm calling the Health Services in Cagliari. Because I'll tell my lawyer about this, about the filth and the dirt. I was in Arno last time, in 2010–2011, and then it was clean, there were people there I got on well with. I've been here with Muslims, and I got on fine with them: they keep themselves clean, even if sometimes they do fight among themselves, in Arabic, not that you can understand very much of what they're saying but they didn't provoke me. I've put all that behind me, I've done the job placement, I passed it and I worked as a gardener for 300 euros a month.

Reflections on Dario's Interview

At the time of the interview, Dario was forty-seven years old, a Sardinian with a great passion for the sea. The sea means freedom, a life free of commitments, infinite horizons. Sometimes it is calm and welcoming, sometimes stormy and unpredictable. It provides sustenance, and Dario, when he wakes lulled by the sea and lifts his nets, is a skilled fisherman.

However, something has wounded Dario, has distressed and agitated him since adolescence, "when you can't figure out what you're doing here". Today adolescence, that difficult and problematic stage in our development, is increasingly frequently the object of psychiatric research as it is now understood that many disorders begin in this period and, if identified in time, can be successfully treated.[11] Indeed, he says that he was being treated by a psychoanalyst because he had a "problem". He points out that his parents have had little formal education and were unable to understand his questions, but then notes that he himself only studied until the third year of middle school. He says he takes lithium salts that "you get from fruit but I need more… no, it's not that I need more, it's that I don't assimilate it". The dosage is 150 mg in the morning and 150 mg in the evening. The tone he uses to talk about his symptoms and treatment seems to indicate that he has little awareness of his disorder (a bipolar disorder?). When he was twenty-one, his girlfriend of the time decided to abort, probably against his wishes.

His first experience of a FPH is in Aversa, after he had smashed up two cars with a baseball bat because the owners insisted on parking in his

[11] Frigerio, A., Rucci, P., Goodman, R., Ammaniti, M., Carlet, O., Cavolina, P., De Girolamo, G., Lenti, C., Lucarelli, L., Mani, E., Martinuzzi, A., Micali, N., Milone, A., Morosini, P., Muratori, F., Nardocci, F., Pastore, V., Polidori, G., Tullini, A., Vanzin, L., … Molteni, M. (2009). Prevalence and correlates of mental disorders among adolescents in Italy: the PrISMA study. *European child & adolescent psychiatry*, *18*(4), 217–226. https://doi.org/10.1007/s00787-008-0720-x.

private parking spaces. He said he had been in all the wards, including the infamous 8bis Cutolo escaped from in 1978 and the Staccata (the ward with the worst living conditions, where violent or agitated patients were confined for long periods on restraint beds).[12] He even did a stretch in the experimental ward without guards. After Aversa he spent a period of time in a Rehabilitation Center in Sardinia and there he has memories of working outside in the fields and the greenhouses. Then he was transferred to the Montelupo Fiorentino FPH. The crimes he talks about and for which he was sent to the Rehab Center (and not to prison, much to his disgust) and then to the FPH were two cases of stalking, involving his ex-girlfriend who he apparently saw after many years of separation and an educator with whom he had a relationship that she rejected, to protect her children.

According to a 2012 study published in the journal *Aggression and Violent Behavior*, "Stalking is generally defined as an intentional pattern of repeated intrusive and intimidating behaviors toward a specific person that causes the target to feel harassed, threatened, and fearful, or that a reasonable person would regard as being so. Motivations for stalking include a delusional belief in romantic destiny, a desire to reclaim a prior relationship, a sadistic urge to torment the victim, or a psychotic overidentification with the victim and the desire to replace him or her. Stalkers may carry a variety of diagnostic labels, including psychotic disorders, delusional disorders, or cluster-B personality disorders, and are generally refractive to conventional psychological treatments. Risk factors for violence in a stalking scenario include a prior intimate relationship, the stalker's feeling of being rejected or humiliated, and generic risk factors for violence such as low educational level and substance abuse."

As explained by B. Gargiullo and R. Damiani (2008),[13] in Italy stalking was criminalized only after a number of very serious cases including that of the stabbing of an actress, Theresa Saldana, in 1982, followed by the murder of another actress, Rebecca Schaeffer, in 1989. Prior to these episodes, the term stalking was applied to cases of harassment, obsessive

[12] D'Agati, M. (2021). *O.P.G. Criminal Asylum. Ediz. illustrata.* 89Books.

[13] Gargiullo, B. C., & Damiani, R. (2008). *Il crimine sessuale tra disfunzioni e perversioni. Con schede cliniche di oltre 70 casi.* Franco Angeli.

behavior, and occasionally to domestic violence. It was declared a prosecutable offence in 2009 (Law n. 38, April 23, 2009).

Dario came to the interview in a collaborative frame of mind. He became quite agitated and excited while telling his story and his tone of voice became vindictive. A man who loves the sea, he is not happy in the FPH. He feels he is confined in a *dump*. Above all, he feels he is being punished, he doesn't feel he deserves this treatment. Reflecting on the people with whom he is forced to pass his time, he says he would prefer to be in prison, "I've never seen them write a letter, read, they're not like me, you know? It's different in prison: you've got a life, you can play football, the people there are the same as me, you can play cards… even if it sounds like no big deal… it's a totally different life, I feel I'm being really, really penalized here." What a paradox! Dario dreams of going back to prison because he feels he would be freer there. Could it be that the FPH is not the right place for Dario, who feels out of place given his resources and state of health? Could prison with its mandate of re-education and confinement be more appropriate for him? Or could it be that Dario's version is not completely faithful to reality and he has omitted some relevant information?

Dario's journey through the labyrinth of the institutions and psychiatric care centers is similar to the odyssey that many psychiatric patients face when their illness reaches the full-blown stage and their families and the regional health services have difficulty in keeping it under control. What happens when the patient commits a crime in the throes of a psychotic crisis or gripped by a behavioral disorder acerbated by drug abuse? As we have seen, prior to 2013 they were assigned to an FPH. After that date, there were no admissions or readmissions to the FPHs. Patients who were no longer considered to be a danger to society (according to the decision of the Surveillance Magistracy, acting on the psychiatrists' reviews) were discharged, while those who were considered as still constituting a danger to society were assigned to the REMS (Residences for the Execution of Security Measures). Patients who had almost finished their detention and so were on probation, could be sent to Rehabilitation Centers for *traditional* psychiatric patients. Some prisons, such as the ex FPH of Barcellona Pozzo di Gotto, maintained a *ward for the mentally infirm* for the observation and treatment of prisoners who developed a mental disorder while in confinement, or those prisoners with mental infirmities who would previously have been sent to an FPH and for whom prisons are not equipped.

In the study published in 2018 mentioned in Chap. 1, Corrado Barbui and colleagues compared the organization of the Italian mental health system forty years after the closing of the psychiatric hospitals with organizations in the G7 countries. They found that for 10,000 inhabitants the availability of beds for mental health in general hospitals was 10.95 in Italy compared to 50.6 in the UK, while Italy had 46.41 beds in community residential facilities compared to 2.28 beds in the UK. In the United States, there were 14.36 beds for mental health per 10,000 inhabitants in general hospitals and 22.29 beds per 10,000 inhabitants in community residential facilities. Therefore, compared to the UK and the USA, Italy had fewer beds for the mentally ill in general hospitals but was by far better equipped to care for these patients in community residential facilities. The UK had a greater number of mental health outpatient facilities (4.94 per 1000 inhabitants) compared to both Italy (1.43 per 1000 inhabitants) and the USA (1.95 per 1000 inhabitants).[14]

As we have seen, Italy has a higher number of places available in community residential facilities, which are based on the Therapeutic Community model.

The term, Therapeutic Community, was first used in the UK in the 1940s; working at the Hollymoor Hospital[15] in Northfield, Colonel John Rickman and Major Wilfred Bion adopted group psychotherapy to treat traumatic neurosis in soldiers returning from the war. However their work had a mixed reception from psychiatrists and from their military superiors and they were forced to abandon the experiment after six weeks. A second experiment was conducted at Northfield by Siegmund Foulkes, in which Tom F. Main, a psychoanalyst participated; he attempted to reproduce the results obtained in the first experiment, limiting the less successful aspects and introducing an innovative vision of the hospital as an organization. He wrote, "The Northfield Experiment is an attempt to

[14] Barbui, C., Papola, D., & Saraceno, B. (2018b). Forty years without mental hospitals in Italy. *International Journal of Mental Health Systems, 12*(1). https://doi.org/10.1186/s13033-018-0223-1.

[15] In 1940, Hollymoor Hospital was converted to a military hospital and was known as Northfield Military Hospital.

use a hospital not as an organization run by doctors in the interests of their own greater technical efficiency, but as a community with the immediate aim of full participation of all its members in its daily life and the eventual aim of the resocialization of the neurotic individual for life in ordinary society."[16] Contemporaneously, but independently, Maxwell Jones, a psychiatrist of the traditional school with an interest in psychosomatics, ran a similar community experiment in the Merton Hill School annexed to the Maudsley Hospital in London. He observed that soldiers with emotional disorders were able to learn a great deal about their own condition and improved significantly if they were involved in interactions and discussions with the staff. He developed his own democratic therapeutic community at the Henderson Hospital in south London from 1946 to 1959.[17] According to Jones,[18] the salient characteristic of the therapeutic community lies in the fact that it is an open democratic system, in which responsibility for the treatment of the patients did not fall exclusively on the medical staff, but was shared by the patients; in his view the process of transformation should take place in group sessions with a focus on the tensions that arose *here and now* and the sole therapeutic objective should be the reintegration of the patient in the world outside the hospital walls. His methodology was based on open communication, less rigidity in the relations between doctors, nurses and patients, daily meetings of the staff and patients, and numerous activity groups. There was no specific psychotherapy program, although Jones was interested in psychodrama and often invited Jacob Moreno, the developer of this method, to the Henderson Hospital; he also used role playing. As in the Northfield experiments, the emphasis was on the egalitarian and the therapeutic aspects of the community approach.

In Italy the residential communities offer the mentally disturbed day and night outpatient facilities with increasing levels of support from

[16] Main, T.F., (1946). The Hospital as a Therapeutic Institution. (Reprinted from the Menninger Clinic Bulletin, Vol. 10, No.3, May, 1946). https://thetcj.org/in-residence-articles/from-the-pet-archive-the-hospital-as-a-therapeutic-institution.

[17] Jones, M.D. (1953). The Therapeutic Community: a New Treatment Method in Psychiatry. Basic Books.

[18] Jones, M. (1976). *Maturation of the therapeutic community: An Organic Approach to Health and Mental Health*. Plenum Pub Corp.

competent staff and varying levels of rehabilitation. Most of the patients who frequent these communities are chronically ill, in the acute or sub-acute phase of the disorder; the severity of their condition at various levels (i.e., biological, psychological, relational, social) does not envisage the possibility of recovery, but they can hope to achieve, slowly and gradually, a fragile equilibrium. The treatment for these patients is of necessity pharmacological but should not be limited to this. In fact, even for these patients, rehabilitation can be considered a possibility.

What exactly is rehabilitation? The World Health Organization defines rehabilitation as "a set of interventions designed to optimize functioning and reduce disability in individuals with health conditions in interaction with their environment". [...] "Rehabilitation addresses the impact of a health condition on a person's everyday life by optimizing their functioning and reducing their experience of disability. Rehabilitation expands the focus of health beyond preventative and curative care to ensure people with a health condition can remain as independent as possible and participate in education, work and meaningful life roles."[19]

In Italy, certain principles of rehabilitation date back to the beginning of the 1800s with what was known as the *moral treatment*. Particularly worthy of note are the reforms instituted by Vincenzo Chiarugi, a Florentine physician who managed to outlaw chains as a means of restraint and promoted the development of rules establishing more humane treatment of the mentally infirm.[20]

Moral treatment aimed at recuperating persons suffering from mental disorders with educational and occupational programs and contact with the environment. However, the medical profession of the time was permeated with superstition, and there was a deeply rooted tendency to see mental illness as a result of some illicit behavior or crime, or unspeakable passions, that could possibly be treated but only in a specific context isolated from the rest of the world, thus giving rise to the mental asylums.

Therefore, a forerunner of rehabilitation was contemplated in the mental asylums, but in Italy true rehabilitation in psychiatry only came

[19] https://www.who.int/health-topics/rehabilitation#tab=tab_1.

[20] Mora, G. (1959). Vincenzo Chiarugi (1759–1820) and his Psychiatric Reform in Florence in the Late Eighteenth Century: (On the Occasion of the Bi-centenary of his Birth). *Journal of the History of Medicine and Allied Sciences, 14*(4), 424–433. http://www.jstor.org/stable/24620719.

into being after the closure of these total institutions under the terms of Law 180/1978 (the Basaglia law).

When therefore does rehabilitation start? According to Kaplan and Sadock (2003),[21] it starts with the diagnosis. The earlier this process starts, the greater is the probability of forestalling the disability. The diagnosis itself however is not sufficient, as however precise and reliable it may be, it does not provide information about the person, their needs, their world. It is essential that the psychiatrist be aware of and familiar with the patient's history, as the symptom must be considered in the context of that particular person.[22]

This process of getting to know the patient is essential for the psychiatrist to identify the rehabilitation processes suitable for *that* patient.

The psychiatric or psychosocial rehabilitation organized in the residential communities includes interviews with a psychiatrist, pharmacological treatment follow-up, interviews with a psychologist and various psychosocial rehabilitation activities, most of which are held in groups and include theater, drama, art, singing, creative writing, reading, gardening, pet therapy, equine-assisted therapy, gym, cooking, English language courses, laboratory. These activities are usually held on a weekly basis and should be proposed to the patient with a specific objective in view. The psychotic with paranoid delusions and the histrionic megalomaniac can benefit from theatrical activities as the play between the real and the imaginary helps them enter into another dimension and experiment therapeutic effects such as a suspension of the delirium. However, these activities must be chosen with care; theater, for example, can trigger undesired effects.

Creative writing can provide a source of personal satisfaction, liberating themes that are difficult for the patient to express vocally in an interview. Gardening, working in greenhouses or a vegetable plot can stimulate a sense of caring for flowers and plants, from sowing to the final act of harvesting. As this is prevalently a manual activity, it distracts the patient

[21] Sadock, B. J., & Sadock, V. A. (2003). *Kaplan & Sadock's Synopsis of Psychiatry: Behavioral Sciences/clinical Psychiatry*. Lippincott Williams & Williams.

[22] Adapted from the doctoral thesis of A. Giancontieri: *Gruppi e riabilitazione psichiatrica, un'esperienza di coordinamento e progettazione in psichiatria* (Università degli Studi Milano-Bicocca—Academic year 2012–2013).

from obsessive and pervasive thoughts and brings them out of themselves. Pet therapy, which in the case of the mentally ill usually involves donkeys, docile beasts that are content to be brushed, led out for walks, is particularly suitable for psychotic patients with a negative and autistic symptomatology. These patients, who have great difficulty forming relationships with people, benefit from contact with these animals, from talking to them and looking after them.[23] Patients suffering from collateral effects (e.g., obesity, hypercholesterolemia, diabetes, etc.) from the pharmacological treatments they are taking, benefit from sessions in the gym and the positive sensation of taking care of themselves and their body. Assembling electrical parts in the laboratory is a form of ergotherapy, and often is assigned with a view to finding paid employment outside the community.

The common denominator of all these rehabilitation activities is the relationship with the patient to be rehabilitated. There cannot be rehabilitation without the acquiescence of the patient, who must be an active participant in the process. There is an ethical problem involved: the facility with which the patient becomes an object around which a series of activities are put into place with an objective that is shared by patient and psychiatrist. This however tends to negate the subjectivity of the patient, with there being too much focus on *doing* and not enough on the search for an interior transformation; the result is that the rehabilitation takes on the characteristics of a simple training course.[24]

In this possible deviation of the rehabilitation process, the activities become *entertainment*. According to Benedetto Saraceno,[25] "the term entertainment, in the context of mental asylums, alludes to both a pleasurable way of passing the time, and to the act of keeping things bottled up inside. Therefore the mental asylums realized both conditions, oscillating between the stronger form of keeping inside and the weaker form of passing the time."

---

[23] Baron-Cohen, S., Tager-Flusberg, H., & Lombardo, M. (2013). Understanding other minds: Perspectives from Developmental Social Neuroscience. Oxford University Press.

[24] Adapted from the doctoral thesis of A. Giancontieri: *Gruppi e riabilitazione psichiatrica, un'esperienza di coordinamento e progettazione in psichiatria* (Università degli Studi Milano-Bicocca—Academic year 2012–2013).

[25] Saraceno, B. (1995). *La fine dell'intrattenimento. Manuale di riabilitazione psichiatrica*. Etas.

There is a risk that today's psychiatric rehabilitation centers could become copies of the mental asylum model if they aggregate large numbers of patients, their rehabilitation activities are not tailored to the individual and they fall back on lengthy courses of treatment, courses that may even last a lifetime. If on the one hand, Franco Basaglia and his collaborators fought to have the mental asylums closed and substituted with new psychiatric outpatient services, on the other the very nature of the mental illness, its elusiveness, incomprehensibility, and the complexity which makes treatment at home so difficult, in many cases condemns the patient to multiple hospitalizations during the course of the illness, in a certain sense defeating the objective of placing them in a *normal* environment.

Given the difficulties and pitfalls that afflict the residential therapeutic communities in their mission to rehabilitate the mentally ill, it is easy to imagine how much more complex must be the task of those psychiatrists who are attempting to rehabilitate mentally ill patients who have committed a crime.

Pietro R. Cavalleri, Medical Director of the Adele Bonolis Foundation in Italy[26] commented on certain situations in which the rehabilitation is imposed by a court order and posed the question, how is it possible to establish a relationship with a patient under these conditions? How are psychiatrists supposed to "take on" these patients, whose primary concern is their loss of physical liberty, which impedes them from expressing their lack of interior liberty? He goes on to ask, in these circumstances, does "taking on" a patient coincide with treating them? Is there a difference between treating and curing? What is it? A cure can only come about if the desire for that cure is sufficiently stable. In the absence of this condition, if it is not possible to cure the patient, they must still be taken care of. The patient can be subjected to rehabilitation by an act of law. In this case, psychiatrists must prepare themselves psychologically to approach a person who is a prisoner twice over: imprisoned by their own lack of internal regulations and, in certain cases, by a constraint imposed by law, which imposes a sanction. This sanction, in turn, crushes the person and catalyzes all their energy with the result that instead of aiming at a

[26] Adele Bonolis Fondazione AS.FRA, Vedano al Lambro, MB, Italy.

transformation, they fall back on pathological strategies that will shore up their false image of a successful io, being the only way they can live with their failures in real life.[27]

In the light of these considerations regarding psychiatric rehabilitation, what forms of rehabilitation will be available to the mentally ill who have committed crimes and are assigned to the REMS?

Lapo: Substance Abuse

Those Evenings on Television

I took part in *Uomini e Donne* in the 1990s. It was different in those days, you went as a couple; I went with my wife, I married when I was very young, I wasn't even twenty, now I'm forty. She was a dancer. It wasn't easy to make a living dancing: those were the days when go-go dancing was all the rage so she changed and became an entertainer, she was the head entertainer in a series of discos and I managed a PR agency. We toured the country… then they called us from the program. We did the audition and they took us. The episode we were on got high audience ratings, so they called us again and again. Then we broke up. They called again but I couldn't face it. In those days I was doing drugs, cocaine, even during the day. I did use it on the program a couple of times, but I didn't enjoy it, my head was elsewhere although I was always lucid at work. From 1998 on, I opened and ran a couple of night clubs, one was already my family's. Up to 1998 I worked in my family's quarry, then I moved into the world of night clubs. In fact, I'm here because of an incident that happened in a nightclub my father ran, where I was giving him a hand with the management. We had a disagreement, my father and I, after sorting out a brawl. Things got a bit heated, because there were some points regarding the nightclub we didn't agree on; he attacked me (although they say it was the other way round) and I punched him because he offended my mother who died when she was twenty-four

[27] Adapted from Cavalleri, P. (2017). La riabilitazione: prendersi cura del paziente. *Journal of Medicine and the Person*,1,95–97.

from alcohol and cocaine abuse. He knew how to hurt, and *he touched a nerve*. I've done martial arts, and it just came naturally; I punched him, he bent over, but my ring caught him and gave him a nasty cut. I could have killed him but luckily I didn't. He needed twelve stitches, seven external and five internal. I got depressed, and started overdosing again even although I was already taking Methadone and Alcover.

I Saw Things in Delirium Tremens...

I've managed to detox here. I'd been out of prison for a year, and I was trying to get clean, but it didn't work. I've gone without for six years in the past...

I did heroine for about six months, but I don't like it. To be honest I don't like any of the other drugs either. Latterly I took drugs because I was depressed, I took them as anti-depressants. I couldn't even work without them. The same with alcohol. Actually, coming off alcohol was the hardest; abstaining from cocaine gives you more psychological problems than physical. I managed to kick the drink by going to TRIAD (*Trattamento Riabilitativo Integrato Alcolismo e Dipendenze*); I did a bit of everything there, operator, chairman, secretary, I wrote articles for their magazine. I won two poetry competitions in prison, I'm good at writing. I read up about alcohol and drugs, studied them a lot but in the end I set a bad example to the people I'd taught. Lots of them relapsed but I was the first to give in; it's tough kicking the drink, probably even tougher than giving up drugs. Quitting alcohol is more than tough; it's easy to get, it's coming back into fashion with all these happy hours and binge drinking. The last two times I ended up in psychiatry. They sent me there from A&E, because now they don't send you to Medicine anymore. They drip-feed you Valium because the DTs are dangerous. Twice the head psychiatrist told me that, "You should be in the Guinness World Records, I've never seen another person upright with 4.59 ethanol in their system". I usually had 4.09, 4.25 and the last time, 4.59: I had 4,000 cocaine in my blood otherwise I couldn't have stayed on my feet. I've seen things when I've had DT! *Mamma mia*... it's hard to put them into words! Hallucinations... I always see people: sometimes I see my partner who says, "don't drink, don't drink!", even though recently she's gone back to the bottle herself. However, she doesn't have the same problem that I have. I'm a true alcoholic and coke addict, she only did it to keep me company. She can stop when she feels like it, she doesn't go into withdrawal. I shook, I desperately needed a drink. When I arrived here I was taking 35 mg of Methadone, three 10 mg phials of Alcover to be taken three times a day, and a lot of other stuff to fight the withdrawal symptoms. When I've got the DTs I see men, men that seem to want to take me away… Dreams and reality alternate, I always get lost in a desert, once I fell out of bed because I thought I was on safari, and at every hole in the road, buuum… at the end they had to tie me to the bed. Like, I was dreaming but I was awake at the same time… it's hard to explain. I couldn't wake up, I called the nurses, I could feel they were moving me but I couldn't reach reality. I spent some really bad days. Then, slowly but surely… When the crisis eases you have something like fibrillations for a couple of days, then it wears off.

When I came here, I was bloated, I played tennis in C series, up to 2010 I played in D when I had the pizzeria. That was when I was off the drink. Actually, I stopped twice, once for two years and the other for five.

On August 15, 2013, I attacked my father. I got arrested the first time for drugs and dealing in drugs in 2001, then again in 2002, 2006, 2010. I got out on October 24, 2012.

I was a pusher, I was in the business, I did it for quite a while, you know, the world of disco. Actually, I was cleared of the first charge: I had 50 g in the house, but I explained it away because I was in a position to do so then. Before they arrested me, I had 450,000 euros in the bank, not in my name—it was in my fiancée's name, because I had that problem of the disco that went bankrupt. My father put me in the business when I was very young, so I've done quite a lot of things. That time I was able to show them that I had money, I showed them my pay slips as my father had quarries and sold marble; I just said I was a heavy user of cocaine, there were three or four of us that evening so 50 g didn't go far. Then they accused me of importing a kilo of heroin and a kilo of coke, but I'd never done that trip and so there was no evidence and I was acquitted after nine years (April 2010). Now there's a claim for compensation pending because, well, I did time for that, I was on house arrest, three years of mandatory residence… without considering the involvement of the television: everyone thought I was a good guy, a hard worker, even though I was doing drugs it didn't show. I only sniffed at night, in the clubs, during the day I only used it if I'd been up late. Outwardly I was fine: then three squad cars drew up… I lived in the city center…, they seized our cars, they talked about a high-class lifestyle—as if owning a Passat and a house is having a high-class lifestyle! They seized everything. My wife's father is an official, her mother works in contact with the public, well, she's not my wife, she's my second partner, the mother of my daughter whose fourteen years old. They really trashed me. After that, no one trusted me anymore: debt collection, trespassing, a second arrest… a bit of a mess. And here I am.

During the trial they asked my psychiatrist's opinion and he said that I'm not a psychiatric case but that all my aggressivity was linked to drugs. Here however I've been detoxed, it's not so easy to stop taking Methadone, Alcover and the rest of the treatment. I did try once before and I almost managed to, but then I went back to the night life too soon and that's where you come into contact with the drugs. Sure, you can say no sometimes, but then when you come up against the first problem, the first discussion with your father or your partner, there you go again. With drugs and alcohol to hand, you get sucked down into that hell, as an ex-addict you can't control yourself, then in that period I was under the effects of Methadone. Come to that, I wasn't taking it because I was sniffing coke, but because I got addicted to it in prison, the Methadone monkey.

I was on heroin for a bit, eight months, then I stopped for my daughter. It just wouldn't have done. That said, they had me tested and decided that I "had diminished capacity at the time of the crime", not because I was out of it, but because I used cocaine habitually, practically every evening. So I was lucid but not myself: Methadone, Alcover, as well as other drugs and alcohol… That evening I'd have said that I felt fine, but now! Now I'd say that I couldn't have been in me to have done all those things. When you lead that kind of life you always feel normal, lucid, but actually you aren't. *Drugs alter your psyche*. Probably I'd have reacted the same, because I'm impulsive, but maybe I'd have thought it over a bit more. Now I do think things over more, but there's still a lot of work to do…

When all is said and done, I'm an addict: and alcoholics are too, because finally alcohol has been classified as a toxic substance, and I've had psychiatric problems related to addiction. Now I should go to a psychiatric rehab center, so my doctor has had to change the diagnosis. Originally, he had written that my problems of aggressivity and impulsiveness were correlated to drugs, but then he had to change that because effectively, taking into consideration my relationship with my mother, I didn't have an easy childhood, I repressed a lot of things, so they've diagnosed me with a *borderline disorder*. At least, this is what my psychoanalyst says, because my psychiatrist says it's all down to the drugs. It's true that drugs cause psychiatric problems because they alter the brain circuits.

Here There's Suffering All Around You, That Doesn't Happen in Prison

Yes, well, my doctor had to change my diagnosis to get me into this place. Now, I wouldn't go so far as to say I'm a fish out of water here, but all the same… because once I kick the habit I'm myself again. I don't have mood swings. This is where you see the difference between here and prison; here you see people suffering, while in prison life is fairly comfortable. The prison in Massa is full of people of all types, they come and go, they're used to it, they know the ropes, they know how to get out. The atmosphere is different, life is different. Here you have to be careful what you do, how you pass the time, how you talk to people. One day I was attacked from behind, punched; luckily, I was able to block the guy without hurting him, because I could have hurt him if I'd wanted to… but once I did hit back. Here you're dealing with people whose moods change from one minute to another without warning, today they'll greet you with a "Ciao, Lapo!", but tomorrow, when you say "hello, X" they're just as likely to say "Who do you think you are, then? I'm Mr. Y to you!". That's just an example. Then there are people who suffer from total delirium… here there's no getting to sleep at night, right now there's a guy in the cell next to mine who is often delirious. There are times when new people arrive and create hell before the doctors find the right treatment. Before I went to work in the kitchens I was a cleaner, and in the mornings I'd find mounds of rubbish in the corridors, some of the cells would be smeared with turds and awash in urine… now that doesn't happen in prison. It's clean in prison; heaven help you if you're dirty there. Here there are health workers but there are cells, well… *mamma mia*… you need to wear a mask if you want to go in. Here there is a "cell worker" who cleans, but with all the cells there are you can imagine how much he manages to get through. He does a couple of bathrooms every day but there are at least sixty. There is one "cell worker" for three wards. He gives the floors a lick with the mop, but he doesn't have time to do much more than that. I'm fortunate, the people in my cell are all *compos mentis*, we are all clean, we cook, we clean the cell every other day because we hardly ever stay in it during the day. When I was in the observation ward I was with a guy who was always delirious, constantly raving, and even when he was lucid he distorted everything. He called me Lucio, thought I was a prophet, sometimes he would talk about the Gospel and then start swearing. I haven't a clue as to why he said certain things, you can't get into someone else's head, it's *unreachable*. I don't think even his psychiatrist understands him. *This is what life is like here.* There's degradation all around you. I don't mean the place itself is degraded, because they do their best, but they can't do everything. There are prison sentences here that last far too long, many could do rehab in other structures such as group-homes, psychiatric rehab centers, specialized psychiatric institutions, etc. There are people here who have committed crimes, killed their mothers and fathers, and been handed out six-month extensions mounting up to six years. For example, there is a person here, he's really calm, he could go to rehab in another place. He doesn't disturb anyone, wouldn't harm the hair on your head, he keeps himself to himself. OK, every so often he talks to himself, but so would anyone who's done ten extra years with promises of being transferred to a rehab centre. I've been here a year already: it's incredible, they need to speed things up.

I Need to Understand Where the Anger Comes From

I hope they decide to send me to the rehab community tomorrow. I was supposed to be here temporarily for six months while they did an assessment to see if I should go free or be sent to prison, but they only did the assessment after eight months and then they said that OK, my impulsiveness was due to drug abuse, but a part was also due to questions stemming from my childhood: the death of my mother, I lived with my grandparents, my father abandoned me, he only took care of the economic side of things. At fourteen years old I would stay out till all hours and at sixteen I started to drink and take drugs. I grew up looking for transgression and I found it on my own; no one forced me. I had the resources, I paid rounds of drinks for all, in a way I was the kingpin. I don't regret anything I did, because I even built houses, skyscrapers, but it goes without saying that if I'd had a mother or father looking after me I would have acted differently. My father tried to recuperate the relationship when I was sixteen, when he got married to another woman, but it didn't work out. However, going back to the assessment, having it done after eight months is ridiculous.

Here in the FPH I've often told the doctors my story. We're all addicts in my family: my father gambled away four million euros. Officially I've been employed for much of my life by our company that sells marble, but in practice I went from one casino to another, I was the cashier. Before it became a discotheque our night club was a clandestine gambling den. It was there that I was arrested the last time… My mother was an alcoholic and a coke head, my grandmother drank. There have been a lot of problems in my family that have been ignored, and so they've gotten worse, and by suppressing them, a lot of anger and impulsivity has emerged. We're working on this, trying to understand where the anger comes from, why I turned to drugs, I'm starting to learn how to recognize the alarm bells. More than a psychiatrist I need a good psychologist. I don't need Valium anymore: I work, I get tired and sleep, I exercise three times a day, 300 push-ups and 1,400 sit-ups. I played competition tennis for years, even when I was taking drugs because tennis is my life. I even played it in prison. Tennis kept me away from drugs for six years. Then I continued playing when I started taking drugs again, sometimes I'd snort a line between sets.

This place has helped me detox, but it's not a good place to be. I don't feel ready to go home yet, not because I'm scared I'll commit another crime, but because I know myself: you learn by your mistakes. I need certainties, more self-awareness, more security. I need a course of treatment that will help me develop my will power, I've already started on it with a psychologist. I don't want to make any more mistakes; I can't afford to. Before it was different, I knew what I was doing. As long as I could control myself, I enjoyed doing cocaine, like I enjoyed a drink. My problem is that I don't know when to stop. I have to convince myself that I need to find strength within myself. I must work on my will power. If I were to get out now, I don't know if I'd have enough will power to say no to drugs when faced with a problem or a discussion. I prefer to be somewhere that keeps you distanced from drugs and helps you strengthen your will power.

Reflections on Lapo's Interview

White, the color of Carrara marble. White, the color of the drug that ensnared Lapo and ruined his life, together with alcohol imbibed in great quantities. Maybe white was also the color of Lapo's father's hair, the father he attacked one evening while under the influence of the drug, leaving him with a nasty cut that required internal and external stitches.

After a number of years in prison for trafficking in drugs, this attack on his father landed him in the Montelupo Fiorentino FPH. Although he was judged to be of unsound mind at the time of the attack as he acted impulsively under the influence of drugs, Lapo states that he is not a psychiatric case. Actually, his life appears to have been fairly normal, and even successful in parts. He participated with his wife in the Italian television transmission *Uomini e Donne* (at that time in its original talk show version), he worked in his father's mining company, selling marble and during that time ran a night club with him. He also had a substantial bank account (though held in his fiancée's name as he had "that problem of the disco that went bankrupt").

It was however a life lived on the edge of pure folly, lived intensely between night and day, work and play, sustained by drugs. Cocaine, in particular. Cocaine is a natural alkaloid with three main pharmacological effects: it is a local anesthetic and a sympathomimetic and stimulates the central nervous system.[28]

[28] Di Chiara, G., & Imperato, A. (1988). Drugs abused by humans preferentially increase synaptic dopamine concentrations in the mesolimbic system of freely moving rats. *Proceedings of the National Academy of Sciences of the United States of America*, *85*(14), 5274–5278. https://doi.org/10.1073/pnas.85.14.5274.

In 1855, a German chemist, Friedrich Gaedecke, extracted the active alkaloid *erythroxyline* from the leaves of the coca plant, and five years later another German, Albert Niemann, developed an improved purification process and gave the substance the name "cocaine" in his doctoral thesis. There was a great deal of interest in its local anesthetic properties, and in 1862 the German pharmaceutical company Merck started to produce small quantities of refined cocaine. In 1884, none other than Sigmund Freud published an essay "Über Coca" in which he recommended the use of cocaine as a cure for a plethora of illnesses, including addiction to morphine.[29] Its popularity increased exponentially over the years, not only for medicinal purposes but also as a recreational drug due to its euphoric effects and efficacy as a sexual stimulant. In 1984, R.K. Siegel, an American pharmacologist, ran a survey to investigate the types of cocaine use from 1970 to 1983.[30] He identified five main types: experimental (a maximum of ten times throughout the life span), social-recreational (usually consumed during the weekend), circumstantial-situational (four to five times a week), intense (at least once a day) and compulsive (more than once a day). Given how Lapo describes his use of the drug, he would appear to fall into the intense category, i.e., daily use spurred by the necessity of dealing with a problem or conflict, or a stressful situation, or again, of maintaining a certain level of performance. In fact, he says he took drugs almost every evening, "I only snorted at night, in the clubs, during the day I only used it if I'd been up late". He said he used it "on the program a couple of times, but I didn't enjoy it, my head was elsewhere". He said that as well as the cocaine, he was drinking heavily; he was well aware of the potentially damaging effects of alcohol and feared its withdrawal symptoms, much more than the withdrawal symptoms from drug abuse. As Maia and colleagues[31] reported, cocaine users are often drinkers. Taking them together

---

[29] Markel, H. (2011). *An Anatomy of Addiction.* Knopf Doubleday Publishing Group, IBSN: 9780307379818.

[30] Siegel R. K. (1984). Changing patterns of cocaine use: longitudinal observations, consequences, and treatment. *NIDA research monograph, 50*, 92–110.

[31] Maia, A. F. D. S., Martins, F. T., Silva Neto, L. D., Alves, R. B., & De Fátima, Â. (2017). Cocaethylene, the in vivo product of cocaine and ethanol, is a narcotic more potent than its precursors. *Acta crystallographica. Section C, Structural chemistry, 73*(Pt 10), 780–783. https://doi.org/10.1107/S2053229617012852.

extends the sense of euphoria and lowers the sense of agitation and paranoia, due to the formation of cocaethylene, which takes longer to eliminate than cocaine. Given the importance that Lapo himself attributed to alcohol and its potentially damaging effects, I will concentrate here on the epidemiological and psychopathological implications and the treatment concerning his abuse of alcohol.

First of all, what exactly is addiction?

According to the American Society of Addiction Medicine, "Addiction is a primary, chronic disease of brain reward, motivation, memory and related circuitry. Dysfunction in these circuits leads to characteristic biological, psychological, social and spiritual manifestations. This is reflected in an individual pathologically pursuing reward and/or relief by substance use and other behaviors. Addiction is characterized by inability to consistently abstain, impairment in behavioral control, craving, diminished recognition of significant problems with one's behaviors and interpersonal relationships, and a dysfunctional emotional response. Like other chronic diseases, addiction often involves cycles of relapse and remission. Without treatment or engagement in recovery activities, addiction is progressive and can result in disability or premature death."[32]

Dr. Michele Sforza, Italian psychiatrist and psychoanalyst, director of the Centre for the Study and Cure of Psychopathologies in Varese, Italy, in an address to the Centro Milanese di Psicoanalisi, explained addition in these terms: "Addiction (from the Latin addictus = slave) is characterized by the individual's loss of control over their impulsive quest for the substance/behavior and the gratification that the acquisition and quest involve. We know that most people (90% of those who drink and 97–98% of those who gamble) do not drink or gamble to excess and so do not suffer negative consequences. However, there is a minority whose levels of consumption and behavior are pathological, and who are unable to extract themselves from this situation even though they are aware of the negative consequences. How can this craving be explained? In his letter to Fliess dated 1897, Freud linked dipsomania with masturbation. Alcohol serves to conceal something that the conscience considers to be

[32] American Society of Addiction Medicine, ASAM News, Vol. 26, n. 3, 2011. https://www.asam.org/docs/default-source/publications/asam-news-archives/2010s/vol26-3.pdf?sfvrsn=12cd5bc2_8.

intolerable. Alcohol's sedative and disinhibition functions are well suited to denial, minimization, rationalization. It is a mood modifier; if taken in small quantities it creates euphoria, in large quantities it results in depression. Edward Glover spoke of alcohol as a defense against paranoia and psychoses, Khantzian (1985) spoke of it as self-medication. Many other scholars have tried to establish the reasons why so many individuals drink, but they don't explain why some of these many individuals, when they have turned to alcohol for some form of comfort, are then unable to stop. They are hooked against their wishes, slaves to the substance/behavior. In recent years, neuroscience has shown how a pathology of the reward system underlies this self-replicating, self-stimulating and compulsive mechanism. There are two main theories of addiction: the first is based on the studies conducted by Olds and Milner, regarding the dysregulation of the reward system, principally involving the neurotransmitter dopamine and its pathways; the second is that proposed by Panksepp, which describes the function of the seeking/expectation system, one of the seven emotional systems (seeking, fear, rage, lust, care, grief, play, and self): the gratification response stimulated by dopamine comes before the satisfaction of the quest, as a sort of anticipatory craving."[33]

Miriam Sebold and her collaborators introduced a neurobiological approach to addiction[34] using the epidemiological data provided by the WHO: the global figure for alcohol abuse is 4% with over 2.5 million deaths per year. Alcohol causes more deaths than HIV/AIDS or tuberculosis.[35] Why do people drink alcohol, even in limited quantities? It is well-known that even a moderate amount of alcohol immediately reduces stress and produces a sensation of relaxation due to its sedative effect,[36] physiological stimulation (with enhanced performance in motor, cogni-

[33] Panksepp, J., & Biven, L. (2012). *The Archaeology of Mind: Neuroevolutionary Origins of Human Emotions (Norton Series on Interpersonal Neurobiology).* W. W. Norton & Company.

[34] Sebold, M., Garbusow, M., Müller, C., Charlet, K., & Heinz, A. (2014). Neurobiology of addiction. In *Springer eBooks* (pp. 9–38). https://doi.org/10.1007/978-88-470-5322-9_2.

[35] World Health Organization, *Global Status Report on Alcohol and Health 2011,* World Health Organization, Geneva 2011.

[36] Zimmermann, U., Blomeyer, D., Laucht, M., & Mann, K. (2007). How gene–stress–behavior interactions can promote adolescent alcohol use: The roles of predrinking allostatic load and childhood behavior disorders. *Pharmacology, Biochemistry and Behavior*, *86*(2), 246–262. https://doi.org/10.1016/j.pbb.2006.09.024.

tive, information processing tests), lightening of negative moods (such as depressive anxiety), increase in talkativeness, feelings of euphoria and social mixing skills.[37, 38, 39] The capacity of alcohol to rapidly reinforce its intake increases the possibility of repeated consumption, which is a factor leading to excessive drinking.[40]

Hasin and her colleagues, writing about the American population, describe Alcohol Use Disorder (AUD) as a chronic illness with a lifetime prevalence of 30.3% and a current prevalence of 8.5%.[41] A high level of disease burden[42] is associated with AUD.

In their systematic review of the changes made in the fifth edition of the Diagnostic and Statistical Manual of Mental Disorders (DSM-5) to the criteria for alcohol use disorder (AUD) compared to those of the DSM-4, Bartoli and colleagues found that the revised diagnostic criteria (which cancelled the criterion of legal problems and introduced the criterion of craving) seemed to increase the prevalence rates of AUD. They attributed this to "the number of DSM-4 *diagnostic orphans* which are more prevalent than DSM-4 single-criterion alcohol abuse individuals."[43]

---

[37] Ekman, G., Frankenhaeuser, M., Goldberg, L., Bjerver, K., Järpe, G., & Myrsten, A. L. (1963). Effects of alcohol intake on subjective and objective variables over a five-hour period. *Psychopharmacology*, *4*(1), 28–38. https://doi.org/10.1007/bf00429361.

[38] Williams A. F. (1966). Social drinking, anxiety, and depression. *Journal of personality and social psychology*, *3*(6), 689–693. https://doi.org/10.1037/h0023299.

[39] Gilman, J. M., Ramchandani, V. A., Davis, M. B., Bjork, J. M., & Hommer, D. W. (2008). Why we like to drink: a functional magnetic resonance imaging study of the rewarding and anxiolytic effects of alcohol. *The Journal of neuroscience: the official journal of the Society for Neuroscience*, *28*(18), 4583–4591. https://doi.org/10.1523/JNEUROSCI.0086-08.2008.

[40] Heinz, A., Batra, A., Gouzoulis-Mayfrank, E., & Scherbaum, N. (2012). *Neurobiologie der Abhängigkeit: Grundlagen und Konsequenzen für Diagnose und Therapie von Suchterkrankungen*. Kohlhammer Verlag.

[41] Hasin, D. S., Stinson, F. S., Ogburn, E. L., & Grant, B. F. (2007). Prevalence, correlates, disability, and comorbidity of DSM-IV alcohol abuse and dependence in the United States. *Archives of General Psychiatry*, *64*(7), 830. https://doi.org/10.1001/archpsyc.64.7.830.

[42] Whiteford, H. A., Degenhardt, L., Rehm, J., Baxter, A. J., Ferrari, A. J., Erskine, H. E., Charlson, F. J., Norman, R. E., Flaxman, A. D., Johns, N., Burstein, R., Murray, C. J., & Vos, T. (2013). Global burden of disease attributable to mental and substance use disorders: findings from the Global Burden of Disease Study 2010. *Lancet (London, England)*, *382*(9904), 1575–1586. https://doi.org/10.1016/S0140-6736(13)61611-6.

[43] Bartoli, F., Carrà, G., Crocamo, C., & Clerici, M. (2015). From DSM-IV to DSM-5 alcohol use disorder: An overview of epidemiological data. *Addictive Behaviors*, *41*, 46–50. https://doi.org/10.1016/j.addbeh.2014.09.029.

Alcohol played a crucial role in Lapo's story: he described, quite emphatically, how it transformed from a form of pleasure to an addiction. He commented on how difficult it is to give up drinking, probably even more difficult than giving up drugs. "Quitting alcohol is more than tough; it's easy to get, it's coming back into fashion with all these happy hours and binge drinking". He described the terrible withdrawal symptoms, both physical and psychological, that forced him to seek help in the A&E, haunted by visual hallucinations. But above all, he points out that in his case, as in many others similar to his, the substances (in his case, both drugs and drink) served to soothe a psychic disturbance; he used them as a form of self-medication. "Latterly I took drugs because I was depressed, I took them as anti-depressants. I couldn't even work without them. The same with alcohol."

Indeed, as Professor Marc Galanter remarks in his book,[44] "The substances can eliminate pain, at least temporarily. Alcohol relieves anxiety and helps the drinker to forget the day's tensions and worries. Stimulants can help those with depression and the opioids remove all forms of malaise and discomfort, creating a state of euphoria and a sensation of lightness. The role of self-medication is very complex. Take George Vaillant's book,[45] for example. He examined six important prospective etiological studies on the origins of alcoholism, finding only very few relations between the psychiatric difficulties in the lives of the participants previous to the onset of dipsomania in later years."

Vaillant's seminal work points out that in a society where it is very easy to obtain alcohol, the possibilities of becoming addicted should not of necessity be linked to a pathological inclination to it. That said, however, Galanter remarked that:

> Recently there has been a significant increase in substance abuse by individuals with serious mental disorders. This phenomenon clearly indicates that, under particular circumstances, psychopathology can lead to the risk of addiction to drugs. In the United States, at the end of the 1980s, the incidence of drug addiction of psychiatric patients in general hospitals was

[44] Galanter, M. (1999b). *Network Therapy for alcohol and drug abuse*. Guilford Press.

[45] Vaillant, G. E. (1983). The Natural History of Alcoholism.

31% and in state psychiatric hospitals it reached 41%. Edward Khantzian, studying the question of self-medication, discovered that 71% of patients addicted to narcotics had mood or anxiety disorders diagnosable with standard criteria.[46]

In a recent review of pharmacological treatment for dual diagnosis published on *Rivista di Psychiatria*,[47] Mario Vitali and colleagues noted that the results of the Epidemiological Catchment Area study show that 13.4% of individuals addicted to alcohol (compared with 7.5% in the general population) suffered from affective disorders and that 21.8% of patients with mood disorders were suffering from disorders caused by alcohol abuse.[48]

Grant and Harford[49] investigated comorbidity between alcohol addiction and major depression in a sample of 42,800 individuals; they found dual diagnosis in 32.5% of the participants and only 11.2% had a disorder from alcohol abuse without major depression. Finally, H. Ross assessed a sample of approximately 8,000 participants aged between 15 and 64, finding that 28.1% responded to the criteria for mood disorders and alcohol abuse.[50]

Lapo's story, which is packed with details, anecdotes that reveal his life and suffering, contains many elements that point to a combination of substance abuse (mainly alcohol and cocaine, but also heroin and

---

[46] Khantzian, E. J., & Treece, C. (1985). DSM-III psychiatric diagnosis of narcotic addicts. Recent findings. *Archives of general psychiatry*, *42*(11), 1067–1071. https://doi.org/10.1001/archpsyc.1985.01790340045007.

[47] Vitali, M., Mistretta, M., Alessandrini, G., Coriale, G., Romeo, M., Attilia, F., Rotondo, C., Del Sorbo, F., Pisciotta, F., Attilia, M. L., & Ceccanti, M. (2018). Pharmacological treatment for dual diagnosis: a literature update and a proposal of intervention. *PubMed*, *53*(3), 160–169. https://doi.org/10.1708/2925.29419.

[48] Regier, D. A., Farmer, M. E., Rae, D. S., Locke, B. Z., Keith, S. J., Judd, L. L., & Goodwin, F. K. (1990). Comorbidity of mental disorders with alcohol and other drug abuse. Results from the Epidemiologic Catchment Area (ECA) Study. *JAMA*, *264*(19), 2511–2518.

[49] Grant, B. F., & Harford, T. C. (1995). Comorbidity between DSM-IV alcohol use disorders and major depression: results of a national survey. *Drug and alcohol dependence*, *39*(3), 197–206. https://doi.org/10.1016/0376-8716(95)01160-4.

[50] Ross H. E. (1995). DSM-III-R alcohol abuse and dependence and psychiatric comorbidity in Ontario: results from the Mental Health Supplement to the Ontario Health Survey. *Drug and alcohol dependence*, *39*(2), 111–128. https://doi.org/10.1016/0376-8716(95)01150-w.

possibly also anti-psychotics such as Methadone) and mood disorders. This can be construed as an example of the use of substances for self-medication. Talking about the attack on his father, he says: "I got depressed, and started overdosing again even although I was already taking Methadone and Alcover". Usually it's difficult to say which comes first, the depression or the drug abuse, but in Lapo's case the psychic disorder, characterized by mood swings and impulsiveness up to the act of aggression, appears to be in pole position, even though he does say, in the words of his psychiatrist, "I'm not a psychiatric case but all my aggressivity was linked to drugs".

Lapo's suffering goes deep and its roots lie in his infancy, in those distorted family relationships. What kind of relationship could the young Lapo have had with a mother addicted to alcohol and cocaine? His mother died prematurely, his father abandoned him, providing only economic support though he did try to patch up the relationship when Lapo is sixteen. Even his grandmother drank. "There have been a lot of problems in my family that have been ignored, and so they've gotten worse, and by suppressing them, a lot of anger and impulsivity has emerged." Lapo is working on this in the FPH, maintaining that he needs a psychologist more than a psychiatrist. He's trying to work out where the anger came from.

The literature confirms how environmental factors such as social deprivation, isolation and abandonment at an early age can increase the risk of developing psychiatric disorders, including substance addiction.[51, 52] Lapo also mentions that there is a history of abuse in his family medical history. Paulus and his colleagues investigate the possible genetic correlations in a family of alcoholics; they individuated a specific endophenotype that has a low response to alcohol, which means that these individuals would need a higher intake than normal in order to feel the stimulating

---

[51] Heinz, A. J., Beck, A., Meyer-Lindenberg, A., Sterzer, P., & Heinz, A. (2011). Cognitive and neurobiological mechanisms of alcohol-related aggression. *Nature reviews. Neuroscience, 12*(7), 400–413. https://doi.org/10.1038/nrn3042.

[52] Meyer-Lindenberg, A., & Tost, H. (2012). Neural mechanisms of social risk for psychiatric disorders. *Nature neuroscience, 15*(5), 663–668. https://doi.org/10.1038/nn.3083.

effect and therefore would need to consume large quantities in order to feel the sedative effect.[53]

Marc Galanter's comments regarding the substantial differences in susceptibility to alcohol from one person to another is useful here in order to show dangerous it is to generalise:

> The use of substances in the context of an illness takes on a completely different meaning. In the case of self-medication, the unpleasant associations that a patient unconsciously tends to make between the use of drugs and the context of the illness, could nullify the positive effects of the substance once the problem that gave rise to the need to self-medicate has been removed. A patient who associates the use of a substance with a previous episode of mental illness will have a negative approach to that substance and will be more critical of it than others who simply consume it to experience a feeling a well-being.

Lapo gives a perspicacious description of the experiences of the alcoholic, particularly when he talks about delirium tremens, when he saw men, "men that seem to want to take me away", "Dreams and reality alternate, I always get lost in a desert, once I fell out of bed because I thought I was on safari, and at every hole in the road, buuum… at the end they had to tie me to the bed. Like, I was dreaming but I was awake at the same time… it's hard to explain. I couldn't wake up, I called the nurses, I could feel they were moving me but I couldn't reach reality. I spent some really bad days. Then, slowly but surely… When the crisis eases you have something like fibrillations for a couple of days, then it wears off." It is evident that he has acquired a good level of awareness of alcoholism, which can also be attributed to his participation in TRIAD. This is a method of treating alcoholics that was used for this first time in Tuscany in 1985. The acronym reflects the three components behind the treatment: the health professionals with medical, psychological, socio-educational, nursing and rehabilitation competences; the

---

[53] Paulus, M. P., Schuckit, M. A., Tapert, S. F., Tolentino, N. J., Matthews, S. C., Smith, T. L., Trim, R. S., Hall, S., & Simmons, A. N. (2012). High versus low level of response to alcohol: evidence of differential reactivity to emotional stimuli. *Biological Psychiatry*, *72*(10), 848–855. https://doi.org/10.1016/j.biopsych.2012.04.016.

volunteers from the alcoholics and their families (in 10 territorial groups) who assist as operators; the volunteers who direct the territorial groups. The mission is to guide the alcoholics as quickly as possible to complete abstinence from alcohol and drugs through a three-phase course, guaranteeing them psychological support and educational/behavioral stimuli in an environment that facilitates a change in their relations with family and society.[54]

TRIAD is just one of several programs for the treatment of addiction. In the Italy in the 1980s treatment courses in the form of systemic family therapy were set up, designed for the *family of the addict*[55] with two explicative hypotheses: an over-protective mother[56] (or family)[57] incapable of functioning adequately without recruiting a son, whose presence in the family circle appears to act as a stabilizing influence on him and helps him to maintain a dynamic equilibrium; an excessively distant maternal o paternal presence, incapable of taking care of the son and providing him with the security necessary for his development towards independence.[58] As these and other theories regarding substance abuse developed, territorial treatment clinics were set up: CMAS—Centro Medico di Assistenza Sociale (1975), NOT—Nuclei Operativi Tossicodipendenza (1980), SERT (Servizi Tossicodipendenze) now known as SERD (Servizi Dipendenze, including NOA Nuclei Operativi Alcologici). In parallel to these drug abuse clinics, therapeutic communities such as Milan's Cascina Verde started to operate.[59]

The *dual diagnoses* patients that the SERD clinics deal with today are complex cases as the use of drugs often induces or brings to light

---

[54] Bernieri, F. (2008). *Alcol e dipendenze. Disintossicare le relazioni: l'esperienza di un gruppo terapeutico-riabilitativo.*

[55] Galanter, M. (1999). *Network Therapy for alcohol and drug abuse.* Guilford Press.

[56] Harbin, H. T., & Maziar, H. M. (1975). The Families of Drug Abusers: A Literature review. *Family Process*, *14*(3), 411–431. https://doi.org/10.1111/j.1545-5300.1975.00411.x.

[57] Goldenberg, I., Stanton, M., & Goldenberg, H. (2016). *Family therapy: An Overview.* Cengage Learning.

[58] Cirillo, S., Berrini, R., Cambiaso, G., Losasso, D., Mazza, R., Vena, G., & Vinci, G. (1995). Un modello di processo eziopatogenetico trigenerazionale della tossicodipendenza. Parte seconda. Idee sul trattamento. *Ecologia della Mente*, 1, 21–40 (non più disponibile—solo riassunto).

[59] Clerici, M. (1993). *Tossicodipendenza e psicoterapia. Implicazioni diagnostiche e valutazione degli interventi terapeutici.* Franco Angeli.

psychopathological conditions that have long-lasting effects and are difficult to cure. These are *new patients*, in whom the risk of committing acts of violence is exacerbated by the intake of drugs or alcohol. Lapo's account of his addition to cocaine and alcohol reveals the strong connection between drugs and alcohol and violence, even though his social functioning seemed to be well under control. This raises the question of how the *dual diagnoses* patient who has committed a crime should be treated: apart from guiding the patient to abstinence and obtaining, where possible, a remission of the symptomatology, what other rehabilitation objectives should there be? New training courses should be made available to health operators who have to deal with these new, changing psychopathologies caused by the new generation of synthetic drugs[60] that are so much more potent than the original. And how should the rehabilitation clinics accommodate these patients who have committed a crime and are therefore subject to security measures; how will the new REMS classify these patients, and how will they manage to deal with the impulsiveness and lack of emotional control that characterizes them?

Arthur: Listening to the Foreigner

I Left the United States and Came to Florence

I've been here in the FPH since 2010; before that I studied Art in Florence. Art helps me digest things. Look! Even while I'm talking to you, I'm drawing. It helps me to let off steam. See, this is what's going on in my head. Nice, isn't it? Here in the FPH when they need a hand with graphics they come to me. In the coming weeks there's a ceramics course in Montelupo, and I'm going to ask if they accept patients too. My story? I left the States in May 2009 and came to Florence. Very soon after that I got sick. I was so sick that I committed a crime, a really serious crime. I gave myself up to the carabinieri, I confessed and went to prison.

[60] Di Petta, G., & Tittarelli, D. (2016). *Le psicosi sintetiche. Il contributo della psicopatologia fenomenologica italiana alle psicosi indotte da sostanze*. Giovanni Fiore Editore.

Sollicciano. Shortened proceedings. I was there for eleven months. A lot of doctors visited me, they said I was unfit to plead. I was sent here to Montelupo.

In prison I couldn't make myself understood. No one understood me. In America I'd asked for help to get treated, *medication for depression*. The college where I studied asked for my medical records and the treatment. I gave them everything.

Three Psychiatrists and an Interpreter

Here in the FPH, it's better than prison; there, there was no space to talk. It was really very difficult to communicate. In the FPH the first thing they did was to offer me an Italian language course. When I was in prison in Sollicciano I had several psychiatric visits: three psychiatrists came to see me with an interpreter. A priest was in contact with my American family. They spoke on the phone. I can't imagine what it must have been like for my family to have to live with this. My family is standing by me. I'm lucky: I can work, and my art helps me. It's different here compared to the prison. I've more contact with the nurses, the doctors, and the guards. Here, if you need something, or something is wrong, you can tell someone, the staff will listen to you. It's not like prison where there are people who are so ill that… maybe it's not possible to treat people in prison. Maybe it's not anybody's fault. I don't know if it's someone's fault, in prison it's like they don't care what you want…

There are no words to describe what I did; an entire family is suffering for the pain I caused… that won't go away…

I prefer to maintain silence. I can't wait to go back to the States and do a course of treatment there… My objectives are very simple: find a job, even as a gas station attendant… I'm not ambitious … do something very normal that helps me pay my way. Get back into society and live a *normal* life, that's what I want to do. I think it should be possible to do that.

Mental Illness and Stigma

In some cases mental illness can be very serious, it can be treated with medicine, it's a serious condition, you can't just ignore it… it's not something to be ashamed of, it should be seen as an illness and treated as such, it should be destigmatized… much of the disgrace that is associated with mental illness is because people who suffer from mental illnesses commit crimes… someone in Montelupo said to me "here there is the FPH, what more could we ask for?" but what did they mean?

Even in the USA taking medicine is seen as a sort of disgrace, not a weakness. Think about the medicine you have to take for your heart. If you don't take that medicine, you'll have a heart attack. If you don't take the medicine for your head, something might happen. Daparox, Zyprexa, and hypnoinducers. They've reduced my medication since I arrived here. I've been here almost five years now and I like working in the kitchens. *Work opportunity in institution.* I get paid for this, I can buy cigarettes. My room is international, there is only one Italian.

Reflections on Arthur's Interview

Arthur's story, as the stories of Izmir and Felipe, throws light on the problems of the foreigner in Italy, their reception and more specifically, of how they fare with psychiatry in this country.

Arthur, for example, is a young American college student who, it seems, started to suffer from depression and so went to a doctor who prescribed medication. Arthur's college was aware of the problem and had asked for his medical records. Then there was the opportunity of a trip to Italy, to Florence, for a period of studying abroad. Once here, Arthur didn't take his medication regularly and started to have problems, probably aggravated by the new surroundings, and didn't look for a psychiatrist to help him. He committed a crime. He didn't go into detail, but from what he says it sounds as if it involved harming a person, as he says, "an entire family is suffering for the pain I caused". After his arrest, he was confined in the prison of Sollicciano but it was a negative experience: "there was no space to talk. It was really very difficult to communicate". These words reflect the essence of Arthur's suffering in prison. There he was, a foreigner, who speaks little Italian and understands even less, confined in an institution incapable of listening to him. Three psychiatrists come to visit him with an interpreter, but it is a priest who coordinates the telephone calls with Arthur's family. He was assessed as being of unsound mind at the time of committing the crime and so was transferred to the Montelupo FPH where he meets with a different reception. Immediately he is offered an Italian course, and he is able to express himself through his art, "Art helps me digest things", he hopes to attend a ceramics course in the town and he works in the kitchens of the FPH, and so earns a little money. He says, "It's different here compared to the prison. I've more contact with the nurses, the doctors, and the guards. Here, if you need something, or something is wrong, you can tell someone, the staff is available to listen to you. It's not like the prison where there are people who are so ill that… maybe it's not possible to treat people in prison. Maybe it's not anybody's fault. I don't know if it's someone's fault, in prison it's like they don't care what you want…". In Arthur's experience the FPH is a place where people listen to you and treat you. His subjectivity emerges here.

An important element that emerges from Arthur's story is his awareness of his disorder and the importance of the cure. When he was in the States, Arthur had recognised the symptoms of a psychiatric disorder and had sought help. He was given a course of treatment, but then, in Italy, "Very soon after that I got sick. I was so sick that I committed a crime, a really serious crime." He somehow manages to see the link, cause and effect, between the disorder and the crime. At the end of the interview, speaking of mental illness, he recognises the severity and the difficulty of such a condition and the possibility of being cured with medicine, "it's not something to be ashamed of, it should be seen as an illness and treated as such, it should be destigmatized… much of the disgrace that is associated with mental illness is because people who suffer from mental illnesses commit crimes…" coming back to the association of mental disorder and crime. He concludes by mentioning that in the USA, in spite of the advances made in psychiatric medication, he thinks that mental disorders are seen as a weakness and taking medicine is sneered at. He compares the medication for mental disorders with that for heart problems, so classifying it as preventative medicine.

From the clinical point of view, what is particularly interesting in Arthur's case is what triggered the disorder when he arrived in Italy. We know that in the States he was taking medicine for depression, and he himself had sought help. So what happened when he arrived in Italy? Possibly he interrupted his medication because of the objective difficulty of finding a psychiatrist, being in a foreign country and unfamiliar with the language. But what happened in Arthur's mind, when he was faced with a new reality, a *foreign* world?

This American college student was catapulted into Florence, a city of middling size, with its immense cultural heritage, open to exchanges with people from every part of the world. Nonetheless, his initial contact with the city was not easy. Maybe he didn't meet the right people to help him integrate into university life and find his way about town, and it is very likely that the language problem played a significant role in creating a barrier between Arthur and his new environment. He didn't know Italian (he was to learn it in the FPH). This immersion in a culture similar to his own but different, was probably traumatic. So his psychic disorder reappeared in this *intercultural* dimension, stronger and more dramatic than before, maybe characterized by melancholic experiences with a psychotic component, linked to the fact of having left behind his home country, his loved ones. A severe psychopathology that together with the dimension of personal freedom—invalidated by the symptoms but still present—spurred Arthur to commit a crime.

Arthur's experiences, together with those of Izmir and Felipe, led me to think about the question of what it is to be a foreigner with psychiatric problems in Italy.

Foreigners bring with them and "inside" them a whole different culture, with their own personal framework of different experiences, symbology, religious beliefs. Indeed, the studies in various disciplines regarding foreigners and their cultures are legion.

According to many authors, transcultural psychiatry came into being in 1904 in an essay written by Emil Kraepelin following on a trip to the Buitenzorg Hospital in Java, where the German psychiatrist had assessed the incidence and manifestations of a pathology he named *dementia praecox*.[61] The expression transcultural psychiatry indicated the comparative

[61] Engström, E. J., & Crozier, I. (2018). Race, alcohol and general paralysis: Emil Kraepelin's comparative psychiatry and his trips to Java (1904) and North America (1925). *History of Psychiatry*, *29*(3), 263–281. https://doi.org/10.1177/0957154x18770601.

study of illnesses or syndromes or therapeutic strategies in various cultures; however it must be kept in mind that that this study assigned a particular role to western psychiatry, the centrality and epistemological foundations of which were never questioned.[62] An editorial of the *Nouvelle Revue d'Ethnopsychiatrie*, on the other hand, indicated the neurologist Gilles de la Tourette as the forerunner of transcultural psychiatry, as his studies on hysteria in 1885 included comparisons with the symptomatology described by authors from other cultures. De la Tourette maintained that it is only possible to fully understand an illness and identify the appropriate cure in a comparative project.[63]

The leap from transcultural psychiatry as a comparative science of cultures to ethnopsychiatry as a frontier discipline, fuelled by cultural anthropology and ethnology, and the psychological sciences (psychoanalysis in particular) that take into account the notion of culture as well as mental illness, was made by George Devereux in 1961.[64] "He was born György Dobo on September 13, 1908 in Lugoi in Hungary (which in 1918 became Romanian); he chose French nationality, then became an American citizen, a Mohave at heart and of Jewish origin. He was truly of mixed race, a collection of cultural components. He spoke many languages and learned ancient Greek at the age of fifty-five. He left his native land, on the border between Hungary and Romania where there were three linguistic communities (German, Magyar, Romanian), for the United States where he lived with the native Indians on a reserve, passing through Paris and Vietnam on his way there. At seventeen he had to deal with the trauma of the suicide of his older brother, Istvan, an experience that left its mark on his entire existence and brought him face to face with psychic suffering".[65]

---

[62] Beneduce, R. (2018). *Etnopsichiatria. Sofferenza mentale e alterità fra Storia, dominio e cultura.* 47–53. Carocci Editore.

[63] De La Tourette, G. (1990). Étude sur une affection nerveuse caractérisée par de l'incoordination motrice acccompagnée d'écholalie et de coprolalie (Jumping, Latah, Myriachit). *Nouvelle Revue D'Ethnopsychiatrie, 15*, 39–66.

[64] Devereux, G. (1961). Mohave ethnopsychiatry and suicide: The psychiatric knowledge and the psychic disturbances of an Indian tribe. *Bureau of American Ethnology Bulletin, 175*, 1–586. http://hdl.handle.net/10088/15469.

[65] Goussot, A. (2014). *L'approccio transculturale nella relazione di aiuto. Il contributo di Georges Devereux tra psicoterapia ed educazione.* Aras Edizioni. (Our translation).

Devereux' ethnopsychiatry reflects his lifestyle, continuous movement, meetings, exchanges of opinions, and involves many disciplines: "anthropology, psychiatry, psychoanalysis, Hellenism, history of religions started to interact. Devereux' project was to place culture, which is the key notion of anthropology, in a new light and have it react (in the chemical sense) with *the* problem of psychiatry: the distinction between normal and pathological".[66]

The distress generated by intercultural contact is one of ethnopsychiatry's chosen fields. In his introduction to the Italian translation of Tobie Nathan's[67] book on Ethnopsychoanalysis that continues the work initiated by Devereux, Salvatore Inglese comments that this discipline studies the phenomenal configuration of the states of emotive, cognitive, behavioural, and somatic disorders in different cultures, their structural strategies of individuation, denomination and interpretation, the culturally codified material operations of adaptation and manipulation of such disorders. Ethnopsychiatry uses complementary methodology to build on an anthropological and psychopathological platform. In fact, cultures always offer a symptomatologic model, a nosological classification, a specific etiological theory and a codified therapeutic technique.

When Tobie Nathan, who had studied under Devereux, opened the first ethnopsychiatric clinic in the Hôpital Avicenne Bobigny in 1979, he was faced with patients from North Africa, Central Africa, Southern Europe (Spain and Portugal), from the French West Indies, from the French islands in the Indian Ocean (Réunion, Madagascar, Comoro), sometimes, though more rarely, Indians from the ancient French commercial centres such as Pondicherry, Turks, and immigrants from South East Asia (Vietnam, Laos, Cambodia, China). Nathan noted that these immigrants "were only described in terms of a deficiency, a social deficiency in particular, phantasmic deficiency or deficiency in the capacity to process [information]. Actually the ethnopsychoanalytic clinic was

[66] Beneduce, R. (2018). *Etnopsichiatria. Sofferenza mentale e alterità fra Storia, dominio e cultura.* 117. Carocci Editore.

[67] Inglese, S., in Nathan, T. (2017). *Introduzione,* in Principi di Etnopsicoanalisi. Bollati Boringhieri.

created from the transformation of these so-called deficiencies into sources of enrichment and innovative techniques."[68]

Ethnopsychiatric knowledge—and indeed, ethnopsychiatric and ethnopsychoanalytic knowledge as Nathan tends to combine these two disciplines in this context—places psychiatry and anthropology in resonance, comparing their respective epistemologies. According to the model proposed by Roberto Beneduce, the term *ethnopsychiatry* can be applied to psychiatry and psychology in all cultures and not just those of the East and Africa, insofar as they are rooted in specific historical and cultural contexts.[69] If we apply this view to Arthur's story, his case could be interpreted in an ethnopsychiatric light, as Arthur's culture of origin is to all effects and purposes quite different to the Italian culture and so could be investigated from an ethnopsychiatric point of view.

The first point that emerges from Arthur's story is his need for someone to talk to, someone who will listen to him, a need that was recognized and fulfilled in the FPH but not in prison. There can be no doubt that Arthur was tormented by feelings of guilt, anger, shame; feelings that the linguistic barrier impeded him from expressing. He mentions that despite the visits of three psychiatrists with an interpreter, there was no dialogue. His story shows that at that time it could not be taken for granted that Italian psychiatrists would be able to adequately understand the needs of an English-speaking patient. In fact, the FPH immediately arranged for him to have Italian lessons so that he would be able to adapt to the new lifestyle. Once he was able to express himself linguistically, Arthur showed a remarkable capacity for adapting to the new context; he found he was able to communicate with his graphic art, he started to work in the kitchens, he was able to communicate with the operators. In brief, his subjectivity started to emerge. Seen under this light, Arthur's stay in FPH was therapeutic in itself, as it provided him with the possibility of learning a language, of expressing himself through his art, of working, communicating, meeting with his relatives, and taking the correct medication.

[68] Nathan, T. *Georges Devereux and Clinical Ethnopsychiatry*. Translated from the French by Catherine Grandsard. https://www.ethnopsychiatrie.net/GDengl.htm.

[69] Beneduce, R. (2018). *Etnopsichiatria. Sofferenza mentale e alterità fra Storia, dominio e cultura*. 315. Carocci Editore.

This case gives rise to a number of questions regarding the approach of Italian psychiatry to foreign patients. For example, what training should the psychiatrist, psychologist, nurse, educator, social worker, have in order to be able to work efficiently with a patient from a different culture? Do institutes teaching psychiatry as a specialization include courses on ethnopsychiatry? What should be the role of the cultural mediator in psychiatry? Should it be purely linguistic, or should this person have at least some rudimentary notions regarding psychic distress and how it manifests in the patient's culture?

Every day we read about migrants fleeing across the Mediterranean in makeshift boats to escape war and poverty in their country of origin, hoping to find work that will allow them a dignified existence in a European country. Debates continue to rage, both at governmental and public level, about how these people should be provided for. At the time of writing this book, psychiatry had a double role to play in the reception process, that of providing treatment where required and also of monitoring the arrivals. On arrival, the immigrants were taken to the Temporary Reception Centers (*Centri di Accoglienza Straordinari*, CAS) where they were assigned an alphanumerical identification code. They wait in these centers for the territorial commissions to decide for which type of protection they are eligible, i.e. permit for humanitarian reasons (one to two years),[70] subsidiary protection (three years), political asylum (five years).

The wait for the session of the commission alone is traumatic, but the hearing itself can be even more so as the immigrants are required to tell their story in detail. Should this experience cause the appearance of dissociative symptoms, the case can be referred to the ethnopsychiatric services organized by the Department of Mental Health.

Once the immigrant has passed through the Temporary Reception Center the next step is the SAI system (Reception and Integration System, *Sistema di Accoglienza e Integrazione*, formerly known as SPRAR, then SIPROIMI), operated in small centres not far from the city center or in any case well connected to it. These centers offer integrated reception services, in addition to board and lodging; the immigrant has the right to

[70] This permit was abrogated by Decree Law 113/2018, implemented by Law 132/2018, (also known as the "Salvini Decree" or "Security Decree").

information services, accompaniment, assistance and orientation through individually tailored socio-economic programs, and apprenticeships. There is also a specific reception program for immigrants suffering from mental health problems; but at the time of writing there were very few places available, indeed, the reception structure of Milan had only eight beds available for psychiatric patients.

The risk of this system is that real, live people are moved from A to B like inanimate objects, identified only by a bracelet with an alphanumerical code. These are people who have survived hardships, hunger, fear, physical and mental trauma, and they are subjected to what amounts to an inquisition by the Reception Commission, whose task it is to ensure that their stories are true. If the experience of reliving their journey, and the reasons they undertook that journey, reactivate dissociative symptomatology typical of Post-Traumatic Stress Disorder, they are sent to psychiatry, to the ethnopsychiatric services for assessment. If the migrant in the Temporary Reception Center or the SAI shows behavioral anomalies such as an aggressive attitude, fighting with their roommate, attempting escape or self-harm, there is the possibility that an educator will take them to the ethnopsychiatric clinic where the staff will work with them to try to understand the reasons behind these behavioral anomalies. The mission of the ethnopsychiatric health worker is to coax the patient to explain their distress and work with them to restore their sense of identity and subjectivity.

Marco: From the Bronx to the Maelstrom of the Drugs

A Life Between Armed Robbery and Drug Dealing

My story is a bit of a mess. On September 10, 1994, I shot up the first time. I was with a group of friends, "What'll we do? Shall we try heroin?" We had just turned fourteen… that's when it all started. I used to go on armed robberies with my Dad, God rest his soul. He took me to Milan, Venice, in Emilia Romagna… Dad was inside for many years, he was looked up to as a boss, and I was the *son of the boss*, so they always dragged me into the trials. I lost my temper once, I said, "My Dad is dead, basta, leave him out of this!". I'm from the Bronx, the Florence Bronx: they're all Sicilians, Calabrians…

My mother was Sicilian and Dad was from Leghorn. Dad was a builder, he had construction companies, all people like that, rigged contracts, they bought cafés… My Dad always said, "Take care of the family first, then of yourself". He bought land to build houses for us, he left us a lot of things. At that time wolf fur coats were all the rage and he had one, a Rolex and a new white Jaguar each year… his mistress lived in a house five hundred meters from ours… my mother knew about her, sure, he paid the rent. That's the world I grew up in, when I was a boy: Dad was buying cafés, with trapdoors to the bisque below. I worked there between elementary and middle school, I served table, the clients often stuffed 50,000 lire notes into my pockets also because I would do jobs for them like collecting their clothes from the dry cleaners. At fourteen years old I always had about 70,000 to 80,000 lire in my pocket. I lived like a king. At the beginning I went with my Dad to do the armed robberies, later I went with someone else, and finally I went on my own. In fact, all the crimes I've been charged with are armed robbery, I'd just one for pushing drugs in 1998.

In 1998 I was eighteen years old. I went to London for the first time on a job. On the way back I fell in with people who had nightclubs and discotheques in Soho, near Piccadilly. I like raves. I'd up and go, even with people I didn't really know. I got engaged to a girl, just like that. But on the way back there was a blitz, a rat snitched on us. They arrested my fiancée's father, her brother, her mother, and her uncle. My girl's father was the organizer, he bought 150,000 pills a week, he ran a whole neighborhood in Rome, illegally. It was a real disaster for thirty-two families: there were people involved I didn't know from Adam. 1,150 pages of phone tapping, really scary. They had tapped all the phones, they had photographs, the lot. During the trial they asked me, "Why have you got money in your hand in this photo?" and I replied, "I was buying a car". Another time they asked, "Why were you switching rucksacks?" "Because I had clothes that needed cleaned and they were taking them to the laundry". But then, showing me a photo where I had pills in my hand, "And now? How do you explain this?", "No comment". After that I kept quiet: I didn't think they had anything to go on, but … This was in 1998. The trial lasted five months, and then there was the sentence. It should have been four years, but I don't know why, they just gave me two for criminal conspiracy. I had tried to defend myself during the trial, saying that the pills were for personal use, but I knew full well that they were aware of my trafficking. They charged me with pushing 10,000 pills a week. I was under supervision: every time I got off a train, I'd be searched by the railway police, but I was always clean and they never found anything. I had a system: as soon as the train emerged from the tunnel I'd throw my backpack with the drugs out of the window. I had another identical, with only a change of clothes, and it fitted inside the one with the drugs. When I got off the train, my backpack contained only a t-shirt, underpants, and a pair of trousers. One of my men picked up the other backpack with the drugs from the tracks. They stopped me once and didn't find anything, and again after 15 days. I spoke to my father about it and he said, "Stop it now, while the going is good; they're on to you" but I was eighteen years old and felt invincible so I said, "OK, don't you worry about it". Then they stopped me a third time and I realized he was right. They were on to me. When I returned to Rome, I called my friends to send a car for me and went to explain the situation to them. "Oh go on! They're on to everyone! Didn't you realize that? They even searched us, random searches". When there is a suspicion of drugs or arms, the police can carry out a search even without a mandate.

We worked together for years, then one day they came and picked us all up.

In the first degree the sentences started from four years, reduced to two on appeal. The charge of conspiracy was dropped, and I had mitigating circumstances, my age, substance addiction, etc. It was a piece of luck that by that time they had abrogated the law that stated that possession of more than 5 pills was attempted massacre.

Close Encounters with the Cops

I did a year and eight months in the common wing, and I got out in 2002. I kept my nose clean till 2006; I worked, I behaved myself, the carabinieri were relaxed because they saw I was working. But then they caught me on CCTV doing an armed robbery. Actually, we had already done quite a few. The day we were supposed to do this jeweler's', it was all ready. I was at a traffic light and I saw this person on a motorbike, a Yamaha TT, but I didn't take much notice… however I saw him again at another traffic light. Then I happened to notice a full-face helmet on a parked bike; I did a U-turn to go get it and I shook off the Yamaha. Unfortunately, they had put a GPS on my bike. Anyway, I took the helmet and left mine in its place, out of respect. It turned out that they were the ones who messed up: they saw me get off my bike and go into the ironmongers (I went in to buy a cutter). There was a queue, but I cut in in front saying, "Sorry to butt in but I've left a job half done because I need a cutter". I left the shop with this pal of mine and I saw three people coming towards me; I remember thinking, "Oh God, don't tell me they're the owners of the motorbike! But not to worry, even if they are on the heavy side I can do this, I've done boxing". I was just about to get on my bike when this voice says, "Stop, stop! Police." They'd blocked everything. "Get down on your knees!" Me, "I'm not getting down on my knees even for God. I'm here, what do you want?". A girl came up to me, I'd seen her before, actually I'd tried picking her up. I remember she'd said, "I'm engaged", and I said, "So what, I'm not jealous". It turned out she was in the police. She tapped me on the shoulder and said, "Bimbo, you've mucked it up this time". I said, "What do you mean, mucked it up? Mucked what up? I haven't done anything". When they opened the bag, they took it badly. They hauled us off to the police station, the Florentine commissioner for armed robberies was there in those days. We heard him blasting the officers, "So you think these two do heists in banks, post offices, betting shops, game galleries? Well, if you'd waited another ten minutes you'd have caught them red-handed!" He was right, of course; if they'd have waited, they'd have got us red-handed. As it was, they held us there till midnight, then the commissioner came and told us to sign a document and then he'd let us go but I refused. I wasn't for signing any document. So he said, "If you don't sign, you go to jail; sign and I give you my word, you walk free." I talked it over with my pal, and we signed. We were beginning to go into comedown, we needed a dose. Anyway, we walked out of that station, hardly believing our luck.

The magistrate hadn't validated the arrest because there was no proof, all we'd done was buy a cutter. We went free for fifteen days but I soon realized they had tapped our phones; while I was on the phone ordering I heard, "No, not that way". Those were the first smart phones. I threw them away immediately, but then I found bugs in the car; though we never talked about anything like that in the car, I sort of suspected they'd have planted bugs there. We were starting to crash that evening, so I called my contact and said, "Let's meet about one, bring me a hand (5 g) but not the usual one, the other one". But he brought me cocaine, I didn't want cocaine, he hadn't caught on that I wanted heroin. "You can take it back, I want heroin." He said, "Wait here, I'll go and come back. You hang on to the cocaine, it's dangerous to go around with that.". He came back twenty minutes later with the heroine and said, "Keep the cocaine, you can pay me later, I trust you". So we went and shot up, because we were really in a bad way, that got us back into shape and we topped up on cocaine for the rest of the evening. Around 6 in the morning we did a last dose and then off to the SERT where we were expected because we sold Methadone there. In the afternoon I met up with Francesco. "What'll we do? Shall we do a runner? We could go to Spain, my father'll help us out with five-ten thousand euro". But he replied, "What about my son?" "We'll take him along, the kid likes me, he calls me Uncle Paolo, I always give him loads of presents". "But my ex will press charges! You go if you want." But I replied, "No, we are in this together, if the boat sinks, we'll go down together". They were waiting for us to do another job. They didn't think that we were pushing heroin too, they thought we just did armed robberies, so we were able to continue with the drugs undisturbed. We bought the phials from Naples: they cost thirteen euros now, before they just cost eight. We would buy five hundred and then sell them here in Florence for at least forty-five. Get a load of that profit!

Then one day as I was leaving the SERT on my scooter a car cut in front of me. I just about had an accident. "What the f@ck are you doing?" I yelled, then I took a better look. It was the cops. They said, "Everything OK? You clean? You carrying something" and I answered, as calm as they come, "No, no, check me out if you want". After a bit I asked, "Well, I can go now, right?", "No. Get in the car. You're under arrest". Me, "OK, but I've got to take Methadone, they give it to me to take it weekly." All the while my father was waiting for me just off the motorway; he wanted to convince me to leave on my own, leaving Francesco behind. But that wasn't for me. Friendship's important for me, I can't stand bastards.

They arrested me. But in those days I was really into drugs…

I've got three black holes in my brain because of ecstasy. I ate loads of the stuff and I collapsed, my cerebellum overheated. I spent seventeen days in a detox center, I didn't remember anything, I didn't recognize anyone. They were really careful with me. I hadn't slept for five days because I'd stuffed myself full of pills, then boom! Everything went black. I've got this flash of being in the ambulance with my girlfriend, she was crying and the doctors kept saying, "keep awake, stay awake!", and then, boom, total blackout. Then, slowly but surely, with photos, films, videos, I kept getting flashbacks, I had these terrible headaches, I cried with the pain… until I got my memory back.

Then I talked to my mother, she used to be a nurse, I told her to get me out of there. "Don't you see how they treat us here? Tied up…" and after a bit I convinced her to take me home. We had a great party to celebrate. The next morning I took the dog for a walk to go see my friends and tell them what had happened. "That's it, no more pills for you. You can smoke as much as you want, but no more trips!" You can say what you like about punks, and people do, but they're good people, they stuck beside me, they aren't rubbish, they've got a heart. They'd take the food out of their mouths to give it to the dogs. I had to send other people to buy me pills because my friends wouldn't give me them. Often, they would make the others take the pills in front of them and that way they lost clients…

Seven Rehab Centers Wouldn't Take Me

I had a psychiatrist in prison, he saw that I was in a bad way; I foamed at the mouth, in those days I was downing lots of pills and ketamine. He said, "But look at you! Look at the state you're in. I'll send you to the clinic because you can't go on the ward in that state". I didn't want to go. Then he said, "Listen to me, I'll help you do just a few years." I stayed in the clinic for three months, in observation, I cut myself a bit… they kept an eye on me, then a criminologist came and said, "I could say you are 70–100% unfit to plead". "What does that mean?", I wanted to know. "With 100% they'll send you to the FPH for six months but at least you won't go to prison." "Hell, I'm not going to prison, then what?" "You can't drive, you can't leave the country, you have to attend a mental hygiene center." Me, "No, no, come on, I don't want to go through that". So he said, "I'll give you 50%, so the sentence will be acceptable". Less than a week later an inspector came, she'd taken my case to heart. She said, "Marco, come on. You're going to the FPH at last". And they brought me here in 2006, then to prison, then back here. In 2012, I got out thanks to article 199:[71] I still had a month to do in the FPH. I did another armed robbery and they copped me. They got me because of my puffer jacket and my shoes: the only robbery I've ever done in a chemist's. The trial went OK, they gave me three years. Three months in jail then they brought me back here to serve the rest. The magistrate said, "You can go to the FPH for the crime committed in 1998". This is all bureaucracy; I don't understand much. I've been here for two years now. It's a mess, they make promises, but they don't keep them. I was to go to a Rehab center in Pistoia, then no, because I'd been there before and I'd smashed things and beaten some people up. Seven Rehab centers didn't want me: the excuse was that my mother didn't get in touch with them, but that is absolutely not true. My mother took the plane to London to come to see me in jail, no way she wouldn't have gotten in touch with the Rehab people. Now maybe they've found a place in a structure, I should start in September.

I'm still on Methadone, I'm down from 70 cc to 13 cc. I'd like to change to Subutex, it's less painful. In the other FPHs you can get anything, here no. In prison you can get anything. Here in Montelupo, no. Mind you, strange things happen here: for example, once my urine test came back positive for cannabinoids and opiates, but I wasn't taking any and in fact the next day the test was negative. There's lots of drugs in Secondigliano, a few years ago they found a kilogram of marijuana in a

[71] Article 199 of the Italian penal code establishes the so-called *double track* system, i.e., the duration of the period of incarceration is accompanied by a security measure to elide social dangerousness.

cell, hidden in a cavity in the wall. Mind you, when things like that happen, you can bet your bottom dollar the guards are in on it.

This place is a prison, a life sentence. You mess up, you get another six months, then another six, then another year. You can't get out of the place. I should have been out ages ago. During the trial, they put me on house arrest but as I'd beaten up a guard here who'd just come back from five months of sick leave, I got another six months.

Here's hoping all will go well in the Rehab center, but I tend to lose my rag when there are too many people about, but maybe I'll like it and it'll go OK…

Imir: Therapy

I Was a Bricklayer; I Killed My Wife

I've been in the FPH here in Montelupo since August 11, 2004. I committed a murder because I was really, really, unwell: I wasn't able to think like I do now and avoid this terrible crime. When I was free, and I got sick, my brother came from a country in Europe, from Iceland. He begged me to take medicine, but I refused. A few months later, this murder happened. I killed my wife. They took me to prison, but I was very unwell and I wasn't able to react and survive in prison. Then the psychiatrists helped me and I was sent here. Here too it wasn't easy in the beginning, I had difficulty taking the medicine. After a couple of months my doctor convinced me: I started taking the medicine and realised that I felt much better.

I've spent ten years here. This institute is very hospitable: the nurses, the doctors, everyone, they have all been very good to me, it's like being at home with my relatives, because they have been good to me too, they come to the interviews since the beginning. After a year or so I got leave and permission spend it at home. So my relatives have stood by me, my brother, my sister, my mother, my brother in Iceland, they were all worried. Now that I've done this course of treatment, this therapy, my relatives are very happy because I feel I have been born again into society. I feel I can say this from the bottom of my heart, because I was so unwell when I was outside. I've done this course of treatment thanks to the doctors, the nurses, and my family. I hope that soon they'll reintegrate me into society, like they reintegrate everyone that has finished serving their sentence. I had ten years to do and they are almost over. My security measure expires in March 2015. We'll see what happens.

I used to live in a town on the border between Emilia and Tuscany. In 2004 I didn't feel good. I was an alcoholic. It's been a long time since I touched alcohol. When I fell sick my relatives took me to Borgo San Lorenzo, that's where our services are. I rejected the help my psychiatrist and my family offered. I refused to accept treatment. Even when I came here, I didn't want to take the medicine. Then after a couple of months they managed to convince me… then I said, "Damn, why didn't I accept this treatment before, when my relatives told me to?" I realized my family and the others cared for me. But at that time I wasn't myself, and I didn't think like I do now.

I was a bricklayer. I worked all week, sometimes I even worked on Sundays; when I had time off, I went into the forest to tidy up the wood. I worked all the time. It was a very critical moment for me because I didn't come to Italy with the idea of hurting anyone, I came to find a better life, to work. But destiny thought differently, and here I am. I work here too; it'll be ten years in December. Here they helped me, they gave me their trust. I work in the kitchen with all the knives and kitchen equipment; a dangerous person could make havoc here. They set me to work three months after I arrived. I cleaned the bathrooms for the first two and a half years, then I did eight months as assistant cook, then I became the cook myself. I've been cooking for my companions here in the institute for seven and a half years. What happened was a disaster. If I'd listened to my family and accepted the help from my psychiatrist I wouldn't be here now. I'm sure of that.

I Come from Albania But I'm a Catholic

Fortunately in these ten years I've never had any problems with the other inmates. I've been lucky because I'm in a room with easy-going people. I've always had good relationships with the prison guards, because I never tried to get one over on them. Even when I was unwell, I never did anything bad to my companions, to the doctors, or the guards. I took the medicine and that was that. Everything fairly normal.

I'd like to get back into contact with the work I did. I started working in 1992; I worked almost ten years in Greece, then I came to Italy in 2002 and worked until I committed that crime. If there wasn't work, I… the medicine, OK, it helps, but I get satisfaction for life from work.

It wasn't at all easy at the beginning. It was hard, very hard. Then, little by little, I got used to the place, to the rules. I ended up in a structure that takes care of you. The nurses and the doctors respect you. They don't punish you; they respect you, even more than you merit. I can't find fault with anyone for the years I've spent here. I'm lucky in that I've never spent a day in prison. The only mistake I made in my life was taking to drink. I deeply regret having done this and I am sure that I'll never touch it again. Never. Honestly, I came to Italy to work… but what happened, happened.

I'm from Albania, where most people are Muslim: fortunately I'm a Catholic. My name comes from that of a poet my grandfather liked. The priest that was here before, he helped my mother to come here and spend Christmas with me when I was on leave then. She taught me six or seven prayers in Albanese. I learned Italian ones quickly: I did the third year of middle school here, I'm good at reading and I can write quite well. I've learned the prayers and I go to hear mass every Sunday. When I'm on leave I always go to church even if there isn't a mass. I pray and I feel like I've been born again. I believe very strongly in God; I pray every morning and every evening and I feel that the Holy Spirit will help me reach my objective of being reintegrated into society like many others. Praying makes me feel good, I pray for my relatives, for my companions and everyone. There, that's what I wanted to say.

Here I've made friends with an American boy who works in the kitchens with me, he came to study in Italy but like me he had the misfortune to end up here. He's a quiet boy, we're in a room together, and we get on well. Then there's a man from Sri Lanka, I get on well with him too. There's a Moroccan, he's just arrived and he's in the room with us. I like him too. Then there's a man from Tuscany… we are like brothers… we all eat together the Albanese dishes that my sister cooks for me when I go on leave, we have coffee together, we clean the room. We're fortunate to be together like this. I've been with the American and the man from Sri Lanka for a long time, I get on well with them. The man from Tuscany has just arrived. I try to avoid arguments. I've never had a discussion in the room. This is a very good thing for us.

I'd Like to be a Cook and See My Daughter Again

When I get out, I'd like to start work as an assistant chef, through contacts because the restaurants outside are different from in here. I'd really like that, but fortunately I can turn my hand to a lot of things: building, painting, tiling, I don't think I'll have any difficulty finding work. Because I admire work and my family. I admire my daughter very much. She's sixteen. She's in Albania with her relatives. She's fine, she's grown a lot and I miss her very, very much. We haven't been able to keep in touch recently because things between me and my wife's family are a very difficult. They don't want me to have contact with my daughter and that makes me feel abandoned, very sad. I've always loved children. She's a girl now, and I hope that when she comes of age she'll ask for an explanation. God willing, I'll tell her what I've told you, and I'll ask her to forgive me and to have contact with me again. Each time my mother comes, or when my brothers go to visit her, they bring me news of her, and photos. She's fine, she's doing very well at school… before I started getting leaves, my mother would secretly pass her to me on the phone. After two years my wife's relatives found out. It was the Christmas of 2009, I asked to talk to her; they passed her the phone and I said, "How are you?", and she answered, "I'm fine. You take your road and I'll take mine", then she started to cry. I understood then that it wasn't her decision, they'd forced her to say that. She's caught between two fires. I know she hasn't stopped thinking about me, like I think about her. She cried and this makes me feel so bad.

This is my situation, my life. If I'd been able to use my head then like I use it now, all this would never have happened. It's no good crying over the past because it doesn't solve anything. You need to find the courage to look ahead, even if it's not easy and my past will follow me for the rest of my life. There are good times and bad times. I'm fine with taking the medicine, although sometimes I feel a bit spaced out, but I'm not worried, I ask for help right away. I want to finish this course of treatment, because it's not right for a person who is able to work and wants to have a family. You need to look ahead and not be crushed by the past. This place has given me strength, has helped me understand how to face things, how to be a free person.

Felipe: All Those Assaults… Just a Matter of Chance?

I Wasn't Drunk, I Attacked a Moroccan

I arrived in Italy, in Genoa, in 2010. I wanted to study and do the course to become a healthcare worker, even if I couldn't speak Italian very well. While I was studying the incident happened: I saw a Moroccan stealing from an old man, so I attacked him with a stick. That's why they brought me here. Nobody reported me, I was in prison for a month and then here. I had a residence permit and my family (mother, sister, cousins, uncles) in Genoa.

I'd never taken medicines, and I'd never been to a doctor or a psychologist. Here is the first time I've ever taken them. They gave me injections, they filled me with drops: Talofen, Rivotril, Valium. A psychiatrist came to see me in prison, but he just wrote. Then he went away immediately. I asked for another, but they didn't send me anyone. I don't know what the diagnosis was, but I got a two-year security measure. I don't like violence.

There was another episode, a bit similar. I was drunk, I was having a discussion with my sister, and someone called the carabinieri. When I opened the door, these guys, because I don't speak much Italian, they threw me to the ground and started kicking me. I kept on saying I didn't understand, they kicked and punched me hard. I didn't know where to go, which hospital to go to. They had to operate on my mouth.

When I attacked the Moroccan, the carabinieri turned up. One was a nasty guy, the other, the good guy, he knew me, and he bundled me into his car. They looked up my CV on the computer, I didn't have a record, the Moroccan was dirty, he wanted to screw me, he was a thief.

Anyway, I wasn't drunk, I go to the Evangelical Church, I'm a good person, I study, read the Bible. They arrested me after that incident and I went to prison.

Here, the FPH, this is a tough place. I cry sometimes. My family is worried. My wife is in my country, in Venezuela, I miss my kids, my mother. I came here to work; I was a bricklayer. On September 22, I've got a hearing regarding some payments of the company I worked for.

At the beginning I worked, but I don't work any more because my knee hurts after what happened with that carabiniere. I play football sometimes, barefoot because I don't have shoes.

I worked for three months in a residence in Sestri Levante, with the old folk. I liked it, we painted, sang, drank coffee, danced…

6

Forensic Psychiatry In Italy: Places of Treatment

Introduction

A Decree of the President of the Cabinet (*Decreto del Presidente del Consiglio dei Ministri*) was passed in 2008 to initiate the processes and procedures necessary to close the Forensic Psychiatric Hospitals (FPH), which were under the responsibility of the Ministry of Justice. Responsibility for the treatment and rehabilitation of the inmates was then transferred to the Ministry of Health. The iter culminated in 2014 with Law n. 81, one of the objectives being to permit the mentally infirm who commit crimes to benefit from courses of treatment similar to those offered to the general public.

As of March 31, 2015, the FPHs no longer accepted new admissions or readmissions and the patients who were resident at the time in the six institutions of Aversa, Barcellona Pozzo di Gotto, Castiglione delle Stiviere, Naples, Montelupo Fiorentino and Reggio Emilia were gradually transferred to alternative accommodation; when the last inmate left Barcellona Pozzo di Gotto in May 2017, Italy became the first country in the world to close its psychiatric-forensic institutions.

Under the terms of Law 81/2014, therefore, mentally infirm offenders who are considered a danger to society and unfit to stand trial are

J. Santambrogio, *Stories from Italian Forensic Psychiatric Hospitals*,
https://doi.org/10.1007/978-3-031-61129-2_6

entrusted to the care of the National Health Service and, when possible, sent to Residences for the Execution of Security Measures (REMS).

Before proceeding, a few words of explanation of the Italian judicial system and its interactions with the health system may be helpful:

(a) Persons who commit crimes and are considered fit to stand trial, i.e. they understand the meaning of their actions and they *decide autonomously* to proceed with such actions regardless of the consequences, if found guilty are *sentenced to imprisonment* or other forms of punishment if the conditions exist;
(b) Persons who commit crimes but are considered *unfit to stand trial due to mental illness* and in addition are considered to be *a danger to society* as it is highly probable they will commit further crimes, are placed under security measures, *probation*, and are subject to regulations which include courses of treatment organized by the National Mental Health Services. In cases where this probation is considered as not being sufficient to contain the potential danger to society, the magistrate orders the person to be confined with a *custodial security measure* in the REMS.

The REMS therefore are specific structures for patients who have committed a crime and are considered to constitute a danger to society but are *not guilty by reason of insanity* (*NGRI*); they are run by health professionals of the National Health Service (and not by prison guards as in the FPH) and their mission is to help the mentally infirm who have committed crimes achieve social rehabilitation through ad hoc treatment programs.

The REMS are located throughout the country, at least one per region, and at the time of writing numbered 31 with a total capacity of 632 inmates.[1] They have a maximum of 20 beds per wing and are bound to respect the structural, technological, and organizational requisites

[1] Garante Nazionale dei diritti delle persone private della libertà personale—Relazione al Parlamento 2023 (the National Authority for the rights of prisoners – Report to Parliament 2023). https://FPH.garantenazionaleprivatiliberta.it/gnpl/resources/cms/documents/24447ddbb0b3093d479d7da93ebcda98.pdf.

established by the Decree of the Minister of Health published on October 1, 2012.

The regions with the highest capacity are Lombardy (120 beds), Lazio (91 beds) and Campania (68 beds). There has been a substantial reduction, approximately 40%, in the number of inmates accommodated in the REMS compared to the FPHs in 2008.

There are substantial differences in capacity from one region to another, however the national average is approximately one bed per 100,000 inhabitants. It has not been possible to compare either this figure with the other EU countries and Switzerland, as there are no common definitions of what constitutes a "forensic bed",[2] or the social-demographic and clinical characteristics of the Italian forensic population to those of other countries.[3]

A constant source of concern is the growing number of mentally disordered offenders considered to be socially dangerous—currently over 675 throughout the country—who are on the *waiting list* for a place in a REMS. Of these persons, 42 are waiting in prison which, as well as being technically unlawful, is a violation of their right to appropriate health treatment.

A recent decision of the Italian Constitutional Court (22/2022) drew attention to the necessity for all parties involved to find more adequate solutions to permit custodial security measures to be implemented without distorting the spirit of Law 81/2014. There are two principal fronts to this debate, those who support an increase in the number of places available in the REMS and those who maintain that the number of places should be reduced to promote the spirit of the reform, increasing the local resources with the objective of eliminating the REMS.

---

[2] Salize, FPH. J., Dreßing, FPH., Fangerau, FPH., Gosek, P., Heitzman, J., Markiewicz, I., Meyer-Lindenberg, A., Stompe, T., Wancata, J., Piccioni, M., & De Girolamo, G. (2023). Highly varying concepts and capacities of forensic mental health services across the European Union. *Frontiers in Public Health, 11*. https://doi.org/10.3389/fpubh.2023.1095743.

[3] L. Castelletti et al. (2023). Places of care in Italian forensic psychiatry: therapeutic aspects and critical issues in an evolving system. *Rassegna Italiana di Criminologia*, XVII, 2, 141–152. https://doi.org/10.7347/RIC-022023-p141.

Staff

As the REMS are part of the Department of Mental Health of the area in which they are established, communications with local and regional health services are greatly facilitated. The composition of the staff has been established with a document approved by the government and regions (including the Ministry of Health, the Ministry of Justice, and the regional administrations) and comprises 2 psychiatrists, 1 psychologist, 2 occupational therapists, 1 social worker, 16 nurses, and 10 nursing assistants for 20 beds (the maximum number foreseen by law). In every REMS, the staff-patient ratio should be 0.9:1. In addition, almost all the REMS can obtain support for the management of any acute crises of individual patients through the psychiatric wards in the nearest general hospital. As a consequence, restraint has been virtually abolished and isolation rooms are also used infrequently. Admissions to acute wards may be on a voluntary or compulsory basis, granted by the Court of Supervision (*Magistrato di Sorveglianza*) and its duration varies depending on each individual's time of recovery.

The main task of the staff is to work on the treatment and rehabilitation of the patients with a view to creating the conditions for them to enter a local mental health treatment program. In spite of the penal nature of the security measures imposed on these patients, the rooms and common living areas of the REMS are residential in design without the elements that characterize a prison environment, however the residences have surveillance systems controlling accesses and perimeters; these systems are both technological (closed circuit television, anti-climb fences, etc.) and physical (guards). All the REMS have a direct line to the local police force for requesting emergency security interventions to deal with aggressions, escapes, etc.

The rehabilitation therapy pursued by the REMS is based on the principles of clinical welfare governance; they are committed to constant improvement of the quality of the services provided and attainment of elevated standards of welfare, while ensuring that maximum levels of security are maintained.

The 2019 Report

In 2019, the Observatory that monitored the situation following the closure of the FPHs, the functioning of the REMS and the coordination between REMS and the Department of Mental Health sent a questionnaire to all the REMS requesting data regarding their resources and functioning from April 1, 2015 to March 2019.

According to the information provided by the REMS, at the time of responding to the questionnaire 526 patients were present, of whom 10.6% were female, 347 (66%) were subject to definitive security measures, 167 (31.7%) to provisional custodial measures (they were known to be responsible for the crime, but their trial was still under way). 12 patients (2.3%) were subject to a combination of custodial measures.

Since the opening of the REMS, 1580 patients had been admitted, of whom 11.5% were female. 1029 patients had been discharged (of whom 65.1% had come from a FPH). 51 patients had returned to the structure after being discharged (of these 3.2% had come from a FPH). The data from the individual REMS showed that there had been no cases of compulsory treatment orders in 8 REMS, in 11 REMS less than 10% of ex-FPH patients had been subjected to compulsory treatment, while in 5 REMS the percentage was over 10% (within a range from 18% to 38%) of ex-FPH patients.

There was a total of 363 incidents of aggression (23% involving ex-FPH patients), which is a significant number and heterogeneous, involving almost 80% of the REMS. This figure, which includes acts of aggression towards staff and other patients, is much higher than that reported in certain studies to be found in literature (23% compared to a range between 3% and 15%). This could be attributed to the impossibility of distinguishing whether an individual patient committed more than one act of aggression. Four suicides were reported, of which 2 in the same REMS.

The questionnaires showed that 80% of the REMS had collaboration agreements with both the Department of Mental Health and with the offices of the Ministry of Justice and the Judiciary. However, it was evident that there was a certain difficulty in establishing courses of treatment as this had been done for only 25% of the patients within 45 days of their arrival, as required by an official document issued by the State Region Conference.[4]

Several critical aspects were immediately evident; there was a lack both of suitable locations with the characteristics required for treatment and of qualified staff to respond to the increase in the quality of the services to be offered by the REMS. There was also the question of the availability of the local services to permit the use of non-custodial measures, as preferred by the Judiciary in accordance with Law 81/2014.

An article published on a specialized journal, the *Rivista di Psichiatria*, drew attention to a number of important factors requiring action: the need to provide appropriate information to the public; training for staff operating in the sector; a greater focus of the psychiatric services on the forensic population; the stipulation of collaboration agreements with the Judiciary. The article also exhorted an efficacious commitment from the various scientific bodies, particularly those working in rehabilitation and involved in the issues related to the identification of courses of treatment and rehabilitation for the post-FPH era. The new system will need time to settle down and become fully operational. As the reform is still in the early years, the actual requirement for beds for the mentally infirm who have committed crimes is still being assessed and consequently it is unlikely that a solution to the question of the waiting list will be found in the short term.

Patient Profiles

As the FPHs before them, the REMS have to deal with persons having committed a wide range of offences and with many different diagnostic profiles. The offences vary from murder to crimes against property, and the task of developing pathways of care to address such complex and varied, often unmet needs, including comorbidities, is extremely challenging.[5] Disorders relating to substance abuse (mainly cocaine, amphet-

---

[4] The *Conferenza permanente per i rapporti tra lo Stato, le regioni e le province autonome* is a commission that controls the collaboration between the State and the regions.

[5] Scales, K. (2014). Doing what makes sense: locating knowledge about person-centred care in the everyday logics of long-term care. PhD Thesis, University of Nottingham.

amines, cannabis, and alcohol) are particularly frequent. Diagnostic profiles include elements crossing all the axes, including impaired expressions of thoughts, affectivity, self-identity, impulsiveness, precarious behavioral control, and antisocial attitudes. Recovery-oriented treatment in forensic psychiatry is a challenge in any environment. It involves engaging patients based on their own goals and strengths and supporting them in finding meaning and purpose by constructing or reclaiming a valued identity and social roles. They should be empowered to become self-determined and thus actively participate in decision-making and treatment planning. These patients not only have mental health problems and functional impairments, they are also burdened with a history of criminal behavior, violence, sexual offenses, high prevalence of comorbid personality disorders, behavioral disturbances, self-harm, and substance abuse. This obviously limits how far recovery-oriented treatment can be fully applied to forensic psychiatric services.

The main objectives of the treatment, set in collaboration with the patient, include improvement of insight, understanding of the disorder and its effects, reduction of symptoms, strengthening family and services' networks, and ensuring therapeutic alliance. Recently the REMS are reporting an increase in admissions of individuals with heterogeneous criminological and security profiles, often having committed no serious offences, who would appear to be difficult community cases rather than "dangerous" subjects. Most of these patients have high levels of comorbidity, such as substance abuse, intellectual disability, and diverse personality traits. For the majority, a referral to the forensic system is seen by the judiciary and health care workers as a last chance for recovery after a series of unsuccessful attempts at treatment. In these cases the psychiatrists attempt to stabilize the symptoms, creating a favorable milieu to engage in a new therapeutic alliance and care network for a future discharge. For these cases the duration of stay is rarely longer than 2 years, and the turnover of admissions and discharges remains quite high.[6]

Accompanied leaves are encouraged if the risk assessment allows, contacts with family and friends are supported where possible, and in some cases leisure or occupational activities are conducted outside the building.

The average length of stay in the REMS is just under 2 years, and readmission rates are low, around 12%. Indeed, in order to reduce the risk of recidivism, the emphasis is placed on individualized care pathways, including psychosocial treatment. Length of stay is of course a key element when developing a treatment plan for these mentally disturbed offenders, as it must take into account court decisions and the quality of cooperation with the Mental Health Services as well as the results of psychiatric assessments. It is interesting to note that Law 81/2014 states that a patient cannot be held in the REMS for a period exceeding the maximum penalty for the specific crime they committed. This solution was introduced to abolish the so-called *white life sentences* that were frequent occurrences in the FPHs, where patients could be detained *ad libitum* simply with a repeated assessment of social dangerousness that in many cases was not associated with any real risk of recidivism. Moreover, the law stipulates that at the end of a security measure, staff may only apply to the court for an extension should the patient show persistent psychopathological instability. Therefore, the security measure cannot be extended simply due to a lack of alternative accommodation in general psychiatry facilities.

A First Evaluation

A study was carried out with the patients of the former FPH of Reggio Emilia to investigate their psycho-social conditions after two years of rehabilitation in the REMS. It emerged that their perception of their

[6] Scarpa, F. Castelletti, L. & Lega, I. The Closure of Forensic Psychiatric Institutions in Italy. https://FPH.researchgate.net/profile/Inga-Markiewicz/publication/333151843_Complementary_Model_of_Long-Term_Care_in_Poland_as_a_Result_of_the_Political_Transformation_Law_Reform_and_Service_Changes_in_Forensic_Psychiatry/links/5ced1a58458515026a6165db/Complementary-Model-of-Long-Term-Care-in-Poland-as-a-Result-of-the-Political-Transformation-Law-Reform-and-Service-Changes-in-Forensic-Psychiatry.pdf#page=312.

quality of life had improved, attributable in particular to the personal satisfaction of being more independent and freer in their movements. Taken together with the low incidence of hetero-aggressive acts, this would indicate that a process of deinstitutionalization is possible in line with the currently applicable laws. The data collected from the survey showed low levels of psychopathy and frequent occurrences of serious psychiatric disorders, which supports the concept that patients from the ex-FPH can benefit from treatment just as all the other patients of the Mental Health Service. There are however still some problem areas to be dealt with, as for example the suicide rate (2 patients out of 47) and the complexity of certain medications, such as Clozapine and a concomitant depot or off label. Patient discharge and rehabilitation should be carefully planned to limit the risk of suicide in a population known to be gravely psychopathological, which has been confirmed by this study.

The study also revealed a need to constantly monitor the appropriateness of the pharmacological treatment, the quality of life, user satisfaction, involvement of the patient in their recovery project, also using specific assessment tools such as Violence Risk Assessment, and a responsible therapeutic risk-taking attitude.

The concept of therapeutic security [7] (Kennedy, 2002), which systematically investigates the relation between treatment and safety in forensic residences, could be developed and applied to the REMS. The classic framework proposed by the Royal College of Psychiatrists is constituted of 4 macro-areas: the relationship between the patients, the staff, the patients' internal world and their relationship with the external world. Relational security is dealt with in the recently published manual "Raccomandazioni di buone pratiche di riabilitazione psico-sociale per adulti" (Recommendations of psycho-social rehabilitation best practices for adults).[8]

---

[7] Kennedy, FPH. G. (2002). Therapeutic uses of security: mapping forensic mental health services by stratifying risk. *Advances in Psychiatric Treatment*, *8*(6), 433–443. https://doi.org/10.1192/apt.8.6.433.

[8] Semisa, D., Bellomo, A., Nigro, P., Merlin, S., & Mucci, A. (2022). *Raccomandazioni di buone pratiche in riabilitazione psicosociale per adulti*. Giovanni Fioriti Editore. Chapter 4.

Other Places of Forensic Treatment

Following the coming into force of Law 81/2014, it was necessary to find a solution for the following categories: people who became mentally ill before their custodial sentence could be executed (art. 148 of the Italian penal code), people considered to be *mentally handicapped* (art. 111, par. 5, of Presidential Decree 230/00), and finally, those who had been sent to a FPH for an *assessment of their mental health* (art. 112, par. 2, of Presidential Decree 230/00). Consequently, at least one prison in each Italian region has a section known as *Articolazione per la tutela della Salute Mentale (Structure for the Protection of Mental Health)* (ATSM) for such persons. In 2021 there was a total of 34 ATSMs, 29 housing 262 men and 5 for 21 women. They are basically prison wards with the attendance of prison guards, run by the Prison Authorities applying prison regulations with the Department of Mental Health providing qualified personnel, psychologists and psychiatrists, sometimes educators or psychiatric rehabilitation experts. However, there is no standard model for these ATSMs and they are not subject to any specific regulation.

The possibility for these wards to provide mental health care for the inmates depends mainly on the relationship with the prison management, the areas assigned and autonomy of action permitted to the healthcare professionals. It is almost impossible to care for people with severe psychopathologies in prison, so inevitably the staff resort to a compulsory medication order and the patient is transferred to a hospital, with the relative problems of transportation and surveillance. The ATSM are sometimes used as a form of transit point for prisoners waiting for a place in the REMS.

As some authors highlight, there is probably no other field of medicine that is so sensitive to the normative and social background determined by the national culture as forensic psychiatry. Italy, benefiting from its radical reform of mental health care in 1978, can discuss and even apply radical solutions to mentally infirm offenders, and continues to be guided by the proposal to eliminate the REMS in the future, leaving the Department of Mental Health responsible for all treatment and care processes for this category of the population.

In addition to these steps forward, what is truly remarkable today is the possibility, if adequately sustained by resources and public interest, of having a legislative and organizational platform on which to develop advanced and solid care pathways in full respect of the civil rights protected by the Constitution of the Republic, and designed to meet the highest standards of care with the lowest possible restrictiveness, depending on the individual characteristics of the case.

Luca Castelletti MD, Member of the National Board of the SIPRiFo (Italian Society of Forensic Psychotherapy) and of the National Board of the SIRP (Italian Society of Rehabilitation Psychiatry), Former Deputy Director of the Veneto REMS

Franco Scarpa MD, ex Chief Medical Officer, FPH Montelupo Fiorentino, Member of the National Board of the SIRP (Italian Society of Rehabilitation Psychiatry) and of the scientific commission of the SIC (Italian Society of Criminology), Director of the SOC Rehabilitation of psychiatric patients who have committed a crime, Central Tuscany

List of Photographs

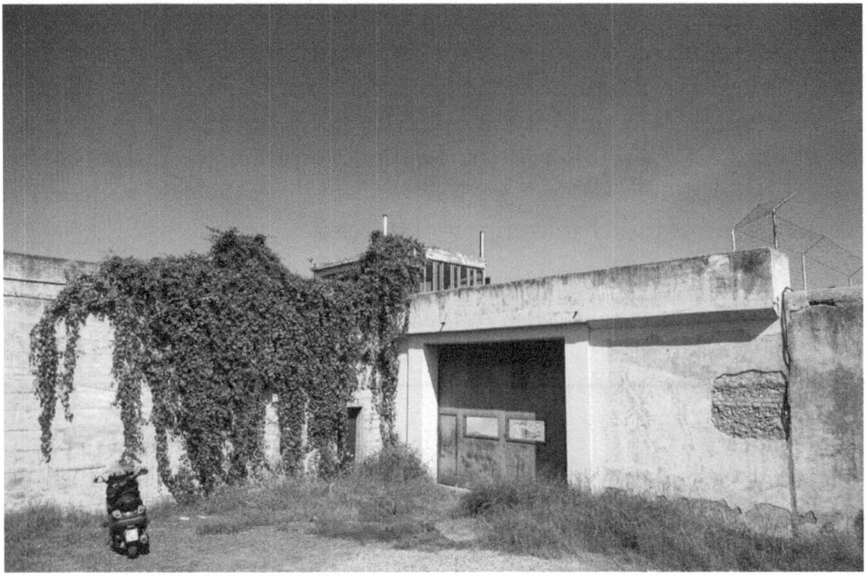

View of the walls of the Forensic Psychiatric Hospital of Barcellona Pozzo di Gotto, 25 September 2013

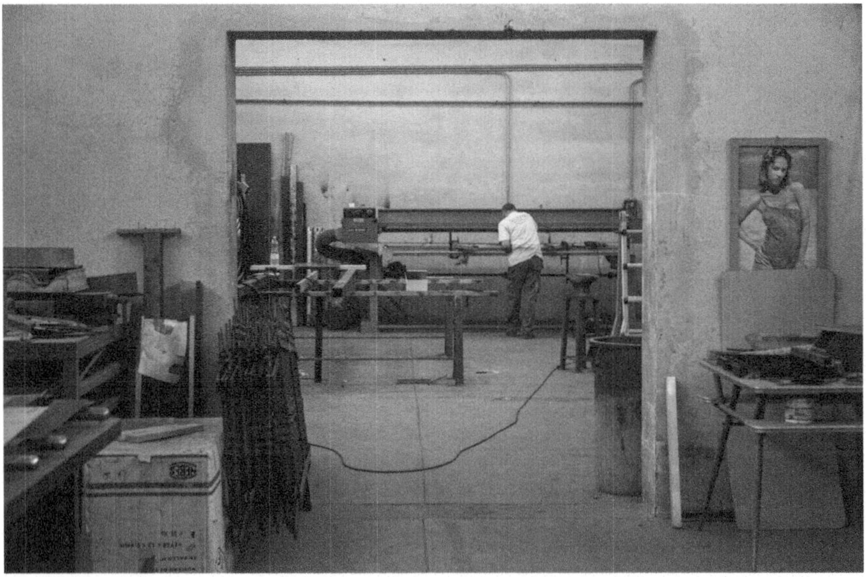

Woodworking at the Forensic Psychiatric Hospital of Barcellona Pozzo di Gotto, 25 September 2013

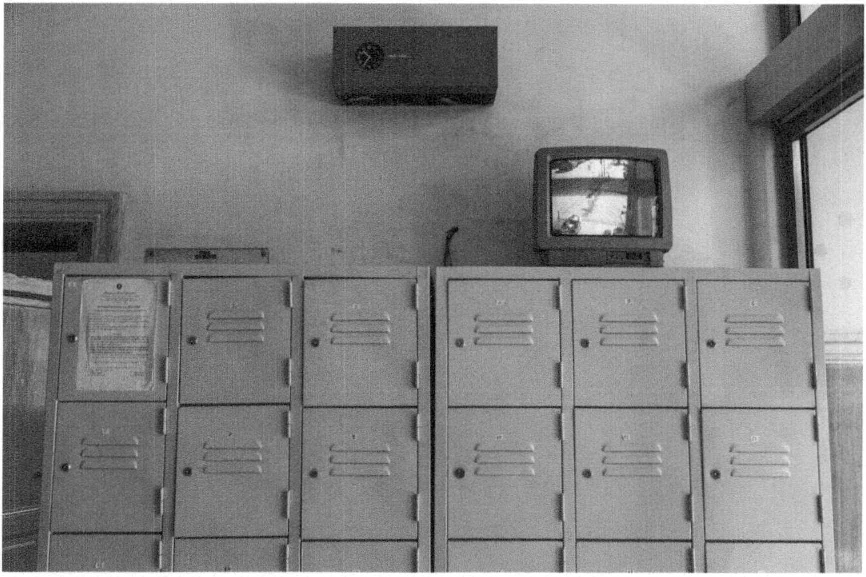

Security camera and lockers in the entrance hall of the Forensic Psychiatric Hospital of Barcellona Pozzo di Gotto, 26 September 2013

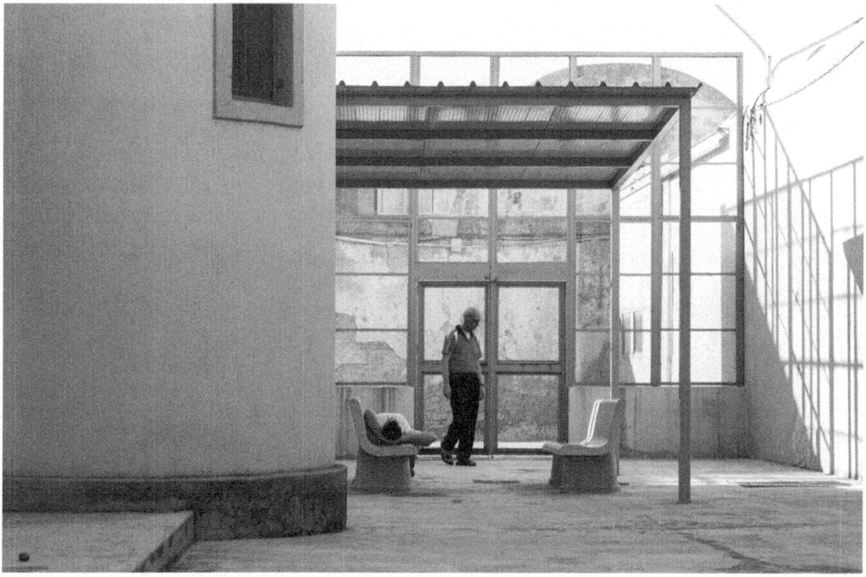

The "walk" and a section of the Forensic Psychiatric Hospital of Barcellona Pozzo di Gotto, 25 September 2013

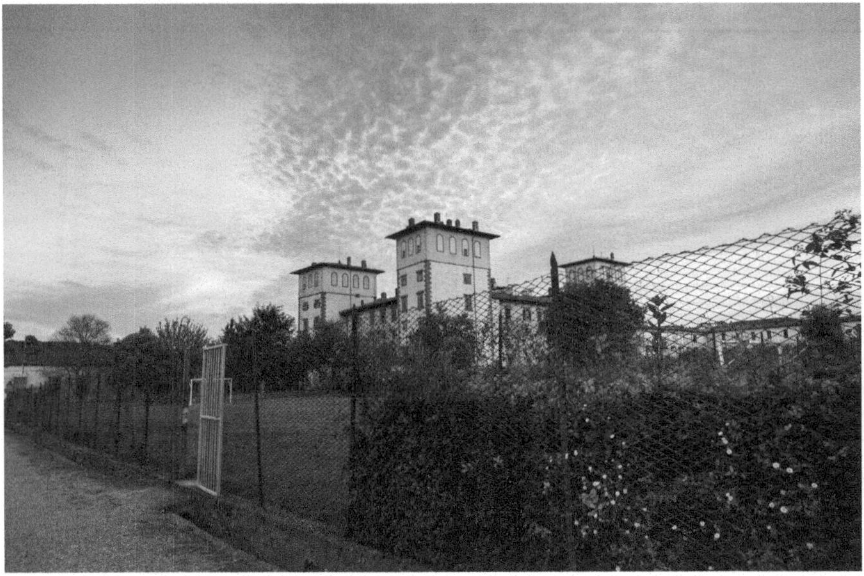

The Villa Medicea dell'Ambrogiana, the Forensic Psychiatric Hospital of Montelupo Fiorentino, 17 September 2014

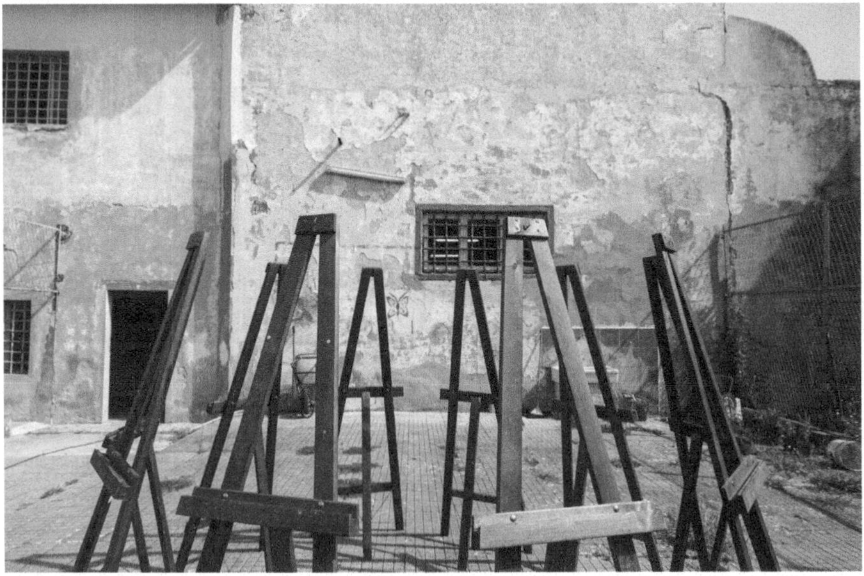

The art lesson, the Forensic Psychiatric Hospital of Montelupo Fiorentino, 18 September 2014

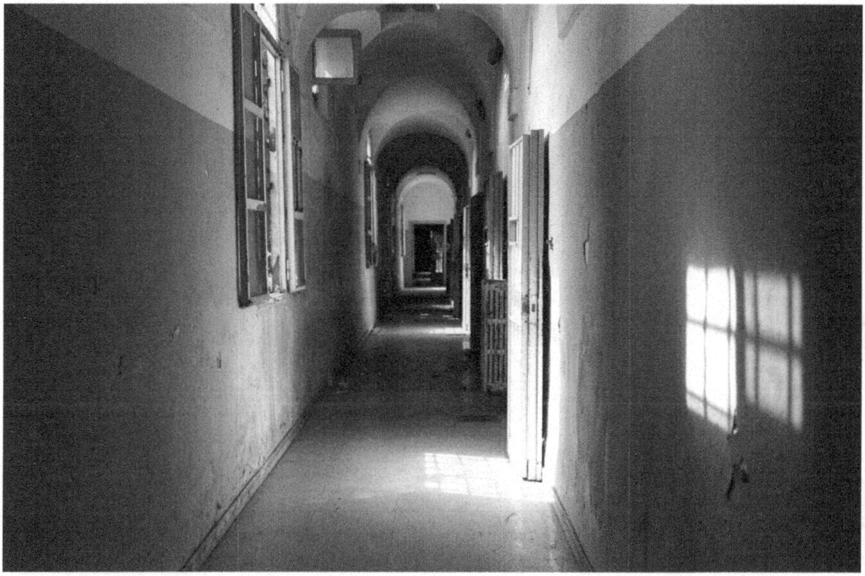

The corridor of the Ambrogiano ward, the Forensic Psychiatric Hospital of Montelupo Fiorentino, 18 September 2014

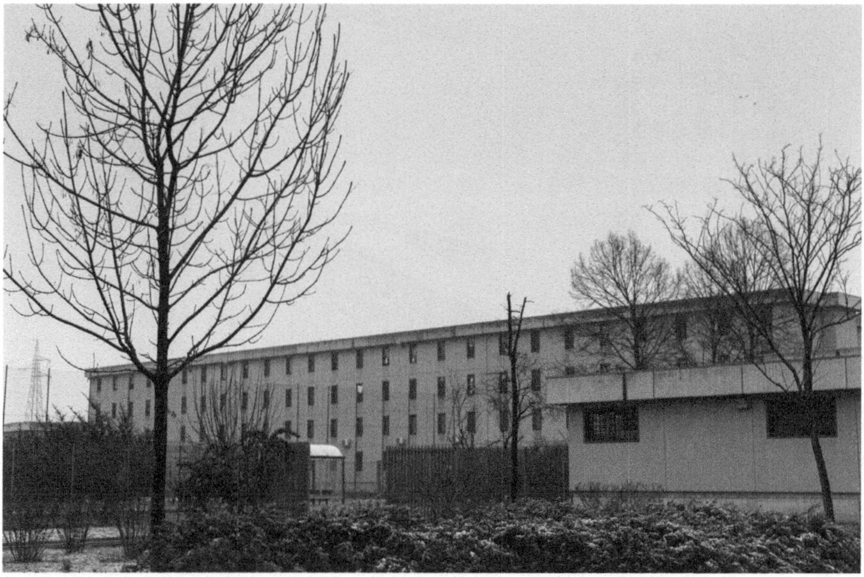

External view of the Forensic Psychiatric Hospital of Reggio Emilia, 28 January 2014

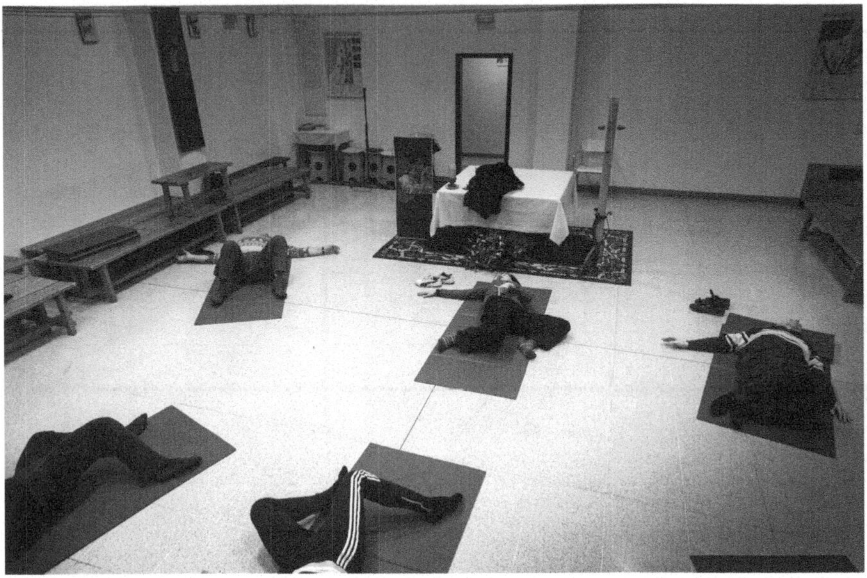

A session in the gym at the Forensic Psychiatric Hospital of Reggio Emilia, 30 January 2014

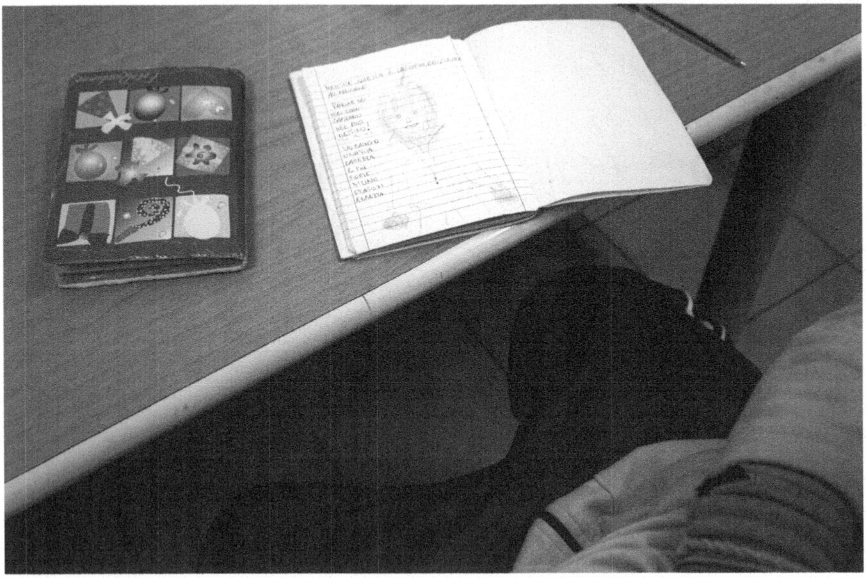

A drawing by an inmate of the Forensic Psychiatric Hospital of Reggio Emilia, 30 January 2014

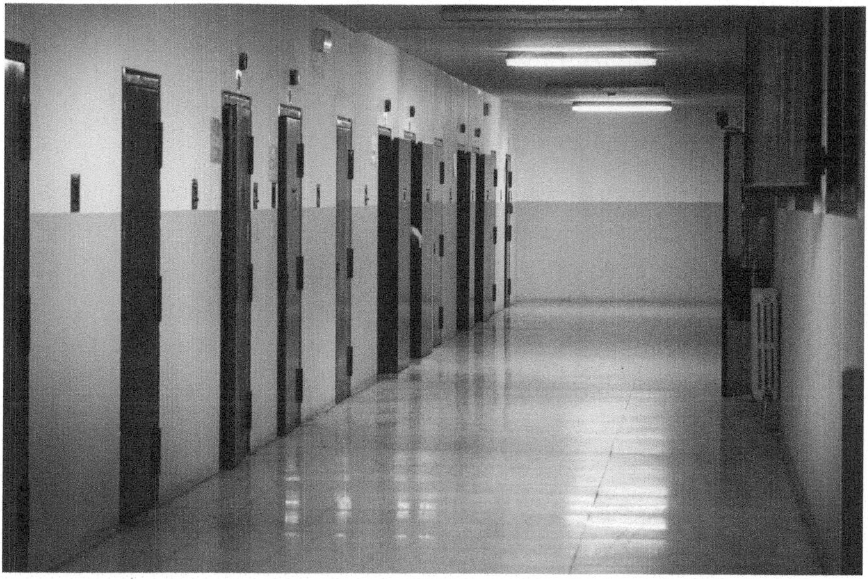

An inmate pushes his hands through the window of a cell in a ward of the Forensic Psychiatric Hospital of Reggio Emilia, 30 January 2014

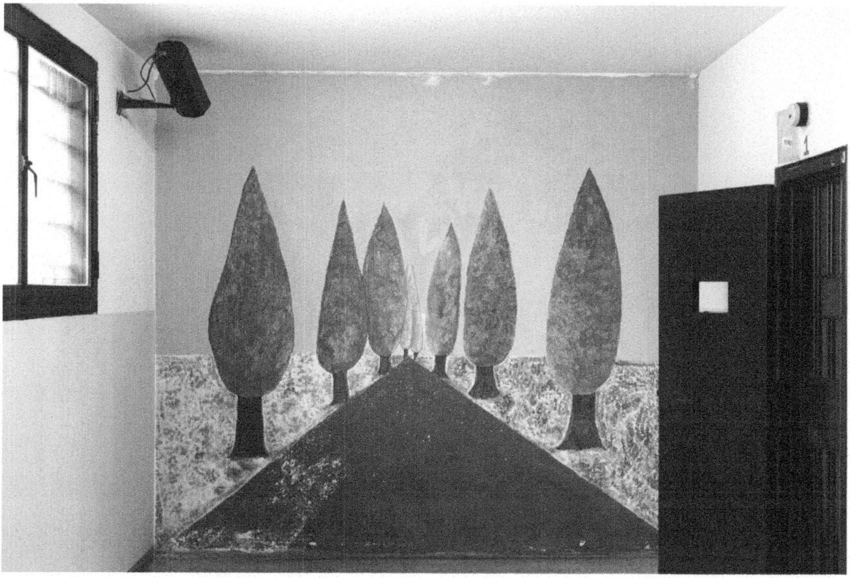

A wall painting in the corridor of a ward of the Forensic Psychiatric Hospital of Reggio Emilia, 28 January 2014

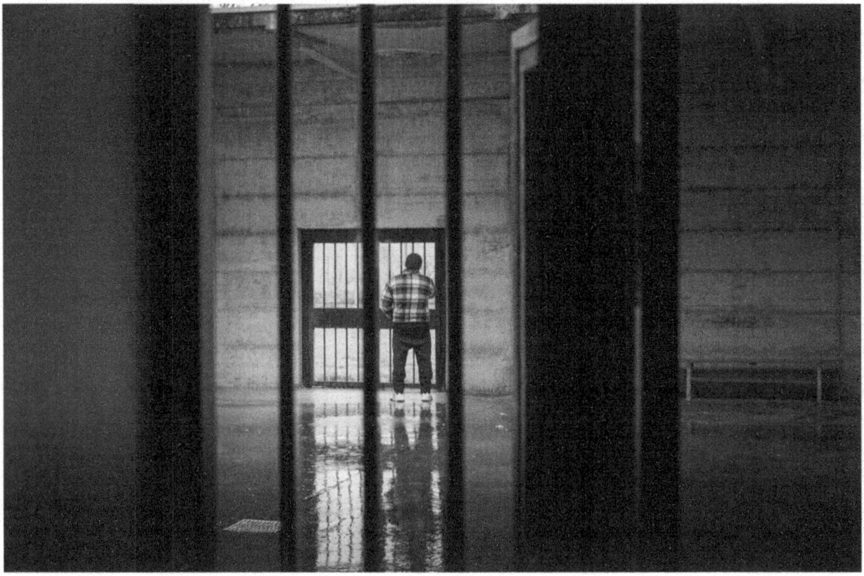

Enjoying the break: the Forensic Psychiatric Hospital of Reggio Emilia, 30 January 2014

Index

J. Santambrogio, *Stories from Italian Forensic Psychiatric Hospitals*,
https://doi.org/10.1007/978-3-031-61129-2

SPRINGER NATURE

GPSR Compliance

The European Union's (EU) General Product Safety Regulation (GPSR) is a set of rules that requires consumer products to be safe and our obligations to ensure this.

If you have any concerns about our products, you can contact us on ProductSafety@springernature.com

In case Publisher is established outside the EU, the EU authorized representative is:

Springer Nature Customer Service Center GmbH
Europaplatz 3
69115 Heidelberg, Germany

The manufacturer's authorised representative in the EU is Springer Nature Customer Service Centre GmbH, Europaplatz 3, 69115 Heidelberg, Germany. If you have any concerns regarding our products, please contact ProductSafety@springernature.com

Printed and bound by CPI Group (UK) Ltd, Croydon, CR0 4YY
01/10/2026
02225967-0011